PHOTO
S0-AXE-720

An aid for the study of Physical Diagnosis

2

G S J Chessell, Dip Ed Tech.
Coordinator, Medical Learning Resources Group,
University of Aberdeen

M J Jamieson, MRCP
Lecturer, Department of Therapeutics and Clinical
Pharmacology, University of Aberdeen

R A Morton, MSc
Director, Department of Medical Illustration,
University of Aberdeen

J C Petrie, FRCP
Reader, Department of Therapeutics and Clinical
Pharmacology, University of Aberdeen; Honorary
Consultant Physician, Aberdeen Teaching
Hospitals.

H M A Towler, MRCP
Lecturer, Department of Medicine,
University of Aberdeen.

Year Book Medical Publishers, Inc.
Chicago

Photo Dix—an aid for the study of clinical diagnosis.

   Bibliography: P.
   Includes index.
   1. Diagnosis—Atlases. I. Chessell, G. S. J. (DNLM:
1. Diagnosis—Examination Questions. 2. Diagnosis,
Differential—Examination Questions. WB 18 P575)

RC71.3.P46   1984   616.07'5'076   84-17350
ISBN 0-8151-1654-3

Printed by Blantyre Printing and Binding Co Ltd

PHOTO D$_X$ — PREFACE

This is volume two of a four-volume series. PHOTO D$_X$ was designed as a study aid to test and improve your diagnostic skills over a wide range of clinical problems.

PHOTO D$_X$ features clinical photographs accompanied by questions that medical students and practising physicians should ask themselves during a patient interview to reach a diagnosis, or may be asked on medical school and board examinations. Answers are provided in a separate section of each volume.

As a part of the continuing education feature of this series, these questions and answers are designed to stimulate additional reading by both medical students and practitioners to further improve diagnostic skills.

The pictures in this new series have been selected from the clinical slide library in the Department of Medical Illustration, University of Aberdeen. The books have been produced against a background of experience gained over the last 10 years in the compilation for local use of over 2,000 self-assessment examples. The local exercise was coordinated through the Medical Learning Resources Group of the Faculty of Medicine, University of Aberdeen, in collaboration with many of the clinicians in the Aberdeen Teaching Hospitals.

The PHOTO D$_X$ series will be of interest to all who are committed to perfecting their skills in clinical diagnosis and to their own continuing medical education. We welcome comment on individual questions and answers.

Although numbering is sequential, each volume in the series is unique, containing a balanced selection of diagnostic examples, and thus may be used independently.

ACKNOWLEDGEMENTS

We wish to acknowledge the invaluable contribution of Dr Anthony Hedley, now Professor of Community Medicine, University of Glasgow, who was the instigator of the self-assessment program on which these books are based. We would also like to acknowledge the cooperation of all patients, secretarial and technical staff, in particular the staff of the Department of Medical Illustration, who have contributed in one way or another to the preparation of these volumes, and Mrs Margaret Doverty who typed the manuscript.

We would particularly like to thank the following colleagues for contributing material for the books:

Dr D R Abramovich, Mr A Adam, Mr A K Ah-See, Dr D J G Bain, Dr L S Bain, Dr K Bartlett, Dr A P Bayliss, Dr B Bennett, Miss F M Bennett, Dr P Best, Dr P D Bewsher, Mr C Birchall, Mr C T Blaiklock, Dr L J Borthwick, Mr P L Brunnen, Dr P W Brunt, Dr J Calder, Professor A G M Campbell, Dr B Carrie, Dr P Carter, Dr G R D Catto, Mr R B Chesney, Dr N Clark, Mr P B Clarke, Mr A I Davidson, Dr R J L Davidson, Dr A A Dawson, Mr W B M Donaldson, Professor A S Douglas, Dr A W Downie, Dr C J Eastmond, Mr J Engeset, Dr N Edward, Dr J K Finlayson, Dr J R S Finnie, Mr A V Foote, Dr N G Fraser, Mr R J A Fraser, Dr J A R Friend, Dr D B Galloway, Mr J M C Gibson, Dr D Hadley, Dr J E C Hern, Dr A W Hutcheon, Dr T A Jeffers, Dr A W Johnston, Mr P F Jones, Dr A C F Kenmure, Mr I R Kernohan, Dr A S M Khir, Mr J Kyle, Dr J S Legge, Mr McFadzean, Dr E McKay, Mr J McLauchlan, Mr K A McLay, Professor M MacLeod, Dr R A Main, Mr Mather, Mr N A Matheson, Mr J D B. Miller, Mr S S Miller, Mr K L G Mills, Dr N A G Mowat, Mr I F K Muir, Dr L E Murchison, Mr W J Newlands, Mr J G Page, Professor R Postlethwaite, Dr J M Rawles, Mr P K Ray, Mr C R W Rayner, Professor A M Rennie, Mr A G R Rennie, Dr J A N Rennie, Dr O J Robb, Dr H S Ross, Dr G Russell, Dr D S Short, Dr P J Smail, Dr C C Smith, Professor G Smith, Dr L Stankler, Mr J H Steyn, Professor J M Stowers, Dr G H Swapp, Mr J Wallace, Professor W Walker, Dr S J Watt, Dr J Weir, Dr J Webster, Dr M I White, Dr F W Wigzell, Dr M J Williams, Mr L C Wills, Dr L A Wilson, Mr H A Young.

195 and 196 This mentally subnormal patient has recently had a first grand mal seizure. The unusual appearance of his finger nail led to close examination of the optic fundi.

a What abnormality is seen in the nail?

b What abnormality is seen adjacent to the optic disc?

c What unusual cause of epilepsy do these suggest?

d What is the risk that his younger sister is also affected?

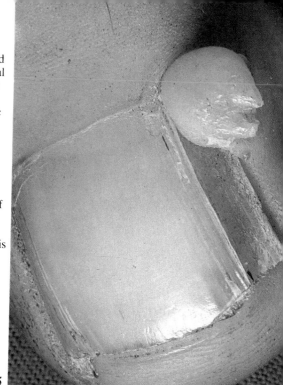

195

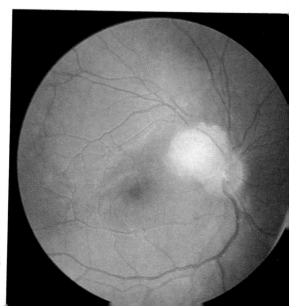

196

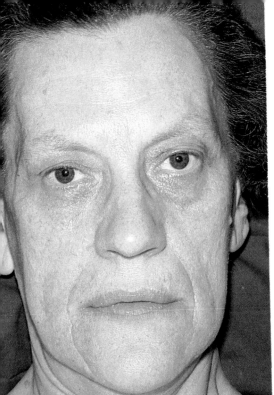

197 This patient complains of tiredness and excessive sweating.
  - a What diagnosis is suggested by her facial appearance?
  - b What treatments are available for this condition?
  - c Which radiological finding is most important in determining the type of treatment employed?

198 This thirty-two year old male presented with accelerated hypertension.
  - a Name the structures labelled 1-5 seen on CT scan through the upper abdomen.
  - b What is the likely diagnosis?

197

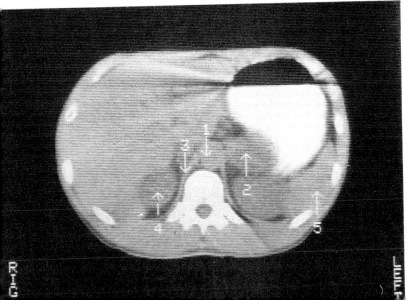

198

199 This twenty-two year old female patient has become increasingly breathless after taking aspirin for period pains.
a What principal radiological abnormality is seen?
b What is the likely diagnosis?
c Is she more likely to complain of difficulty breathing in or breathing out?

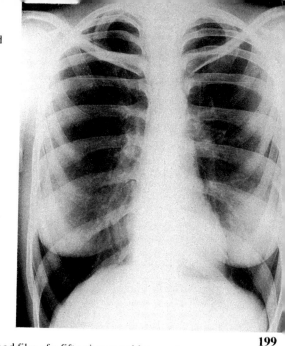

199

200 This is the peripheral blood film of a fifty-six year old man who presented with tiredness and a sensation of abdominal fullness. 15 cm splenomegaly was noted. His haemoglobin was 9.5 g/dl, white cell count $130 \times 10^9/1$, and platelets $600 \times 10^9/1$.
a What diagnosis does the film suggest?
b Name three investigations performed on peripheral blood which may help establish the diagnosis.
c Name four drugs employed in the management of this disease.

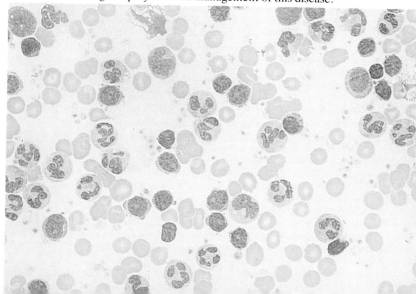

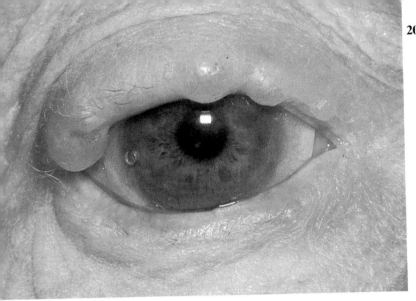

201

201 This woman has ocular cicatrical pemphigoid.
  a What is the main complication of this condition?
  b What would immunofluorescence studies of a skin biopsy show?
  c Is this associated with underlying malignancy?

202 This driver of an
  articulated lorry
  complains of chest pain.
  a What is the diagnosis?
  b When should he return
     to driving his lorry?

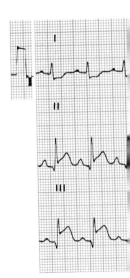

203

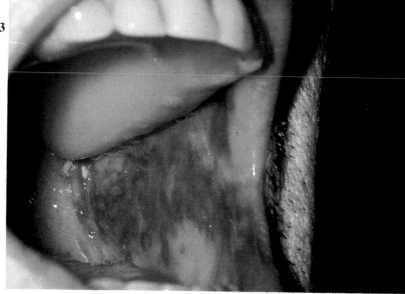

203 This forty-five year old man presented with a short history of increasing muscle weakness, weight loss and ankle swelling. He was unable to rise from a chair without using his arms. His blood pressure was 180/110 mm Hg. sitting.

a What is the likely diagnosis?

b Where is the likely site of the underlying lesion?

c What electrolyte abnormality may be present?

d Which investigations may help establish the diagnosis?

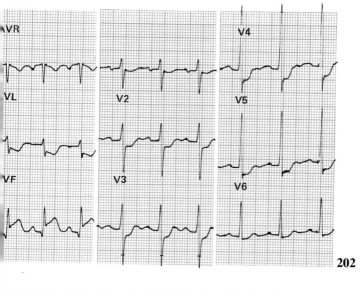

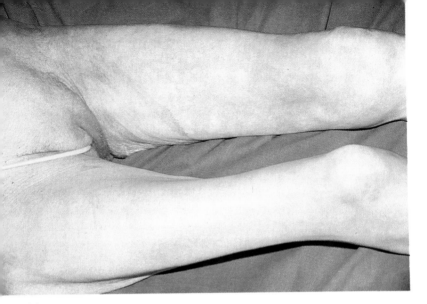

204

205

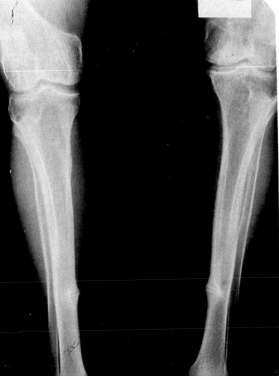

204 This patient has been in hospital for three months following a stroke. She has longstanding mitral valve disease. Four hours ago she complained of pain and coldness affecting her left leg.
   a What is the likely diagnosis?
   b What is the most likely origin of this problem?
   c What disorder of cardiac rhythm would you expect to find?

205 This female patient is a recent immigrant into the United Kingdom from India.
   a What bony abnormali￼ is seen in her x-ray?
   b In which other sites ar￼ these typically seen?
   c What metabolic disorder do these indicate?

206 This patient complains of severe generalised pruritus, worst when in bed at night.

  a What is the most likely diagnosis?

  b In which sites should the causative agent be sought?

  c How is the diagnosis confirmed?

207 This child has always been prone to chest infections. Her height is consistently below the third centile for her age. Recently, for the first time, her fingers have been seen to be intermittently cyanosed. A pansystolic murmur is audible at the left sternal edge. E.C.G. shows tall P waves in standard lead II and dominant R waves in leads V_1 to V_3.

  a What is the most likely diagnosis?

  b Why is she cyanosed?

  c What abnormalities in haemodynamics and in oxygen saturation would you expect to find at cardiac catheterisation?

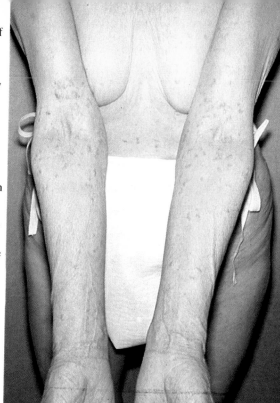

206

207

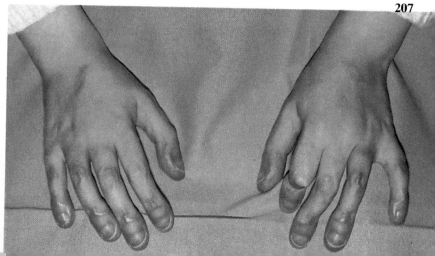

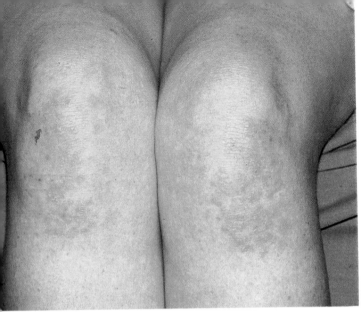

208

209 a What name is given to this infection?
  b What is the infecting organism?
  c What is its usual origin?

209

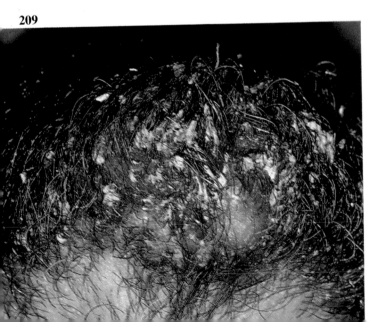

208 This patient complains of an intensely itchy skin rash. On specific questioning she admits to chronic mild diarrhoea, the stools on occasion being difficult to flush.

  a What name is given to the skin rash?

  b What is likely to be the cause of her abdominal symptoms?

  c What two forms of treatment may improve the skin rash?

210 a What name is given to the lesion seen on the right side of this patient's tongue?

  b What is its significance?

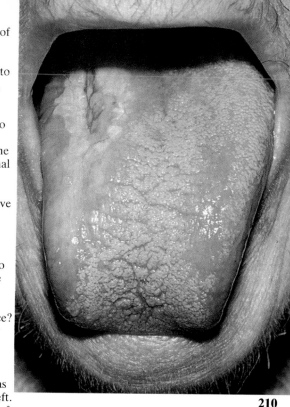

210

211 This Asian patient was asked to look to his left.

  a What abnormality of eye movement is shown?

  b What is the cranial nerve lesion involved?

211

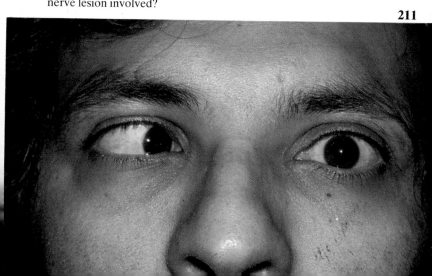

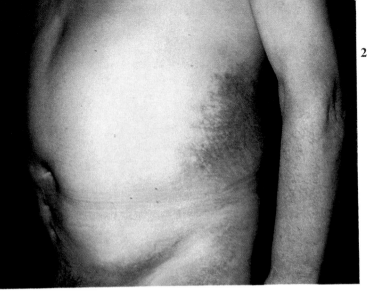

212 This patient presents with acute onset spontaneous back pain.
   a Which two eponymous signs are present?
   b Which diagnoses should be considered?

213 a Which two abnormalities are seen here?
   b What is the most likely underlying disorder?
   c List four other stigmata of this disorder which may be observed in the hands.

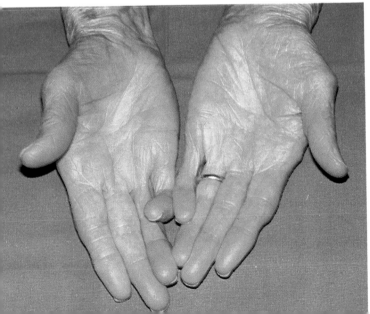

214 This patient complains of sudden visual loss in this eye.

What abnormality is seen in this peripheral area of the fundus?

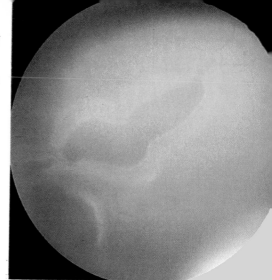

214

215 This male child falls frequently and finds running difficult. There is a family history of similar problems.

a What muscular abnormality is shown?

b What is the likely diagnosis?

c What eponym is used to describe the characteristic manoeuvre by which such children stand up from lying prone?

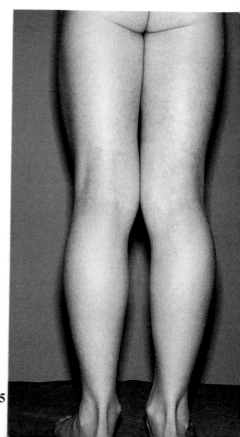

215

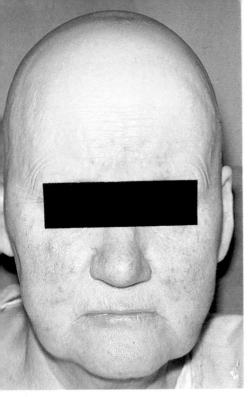

216

216 and 217 This patient has recently developed dysphagia.
a What principal abnormalities are seen in
i) the head?
ii) the hands?
b What is the underlying diagnosis?

217

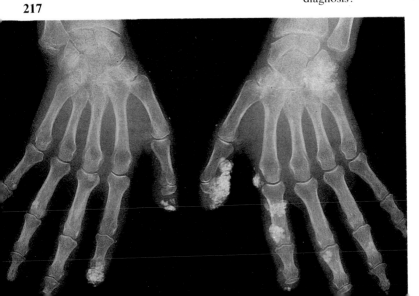

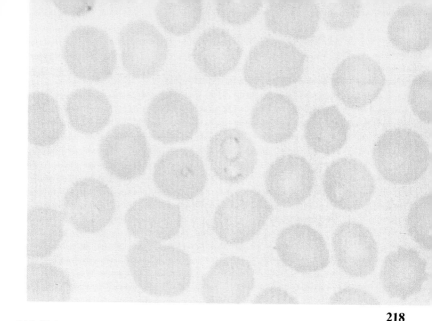

218

218 This oilworker recently returned from Thailand, having taken chloroquine anti-malarial prophylaxis. He complained of fever, headache, and widespread arthralgia.
   a What abnormality is seen on this thin blood film?
   b What immediate therapy is indicated?
   c What prophylaxis would have been appropriate?

219

219 a List four abnormalities visible on this child's intravenous pyelogram.
   b What electrolyte disturbances are typical of the urinary abnormality?
   c Would you expect to find an anion gap?

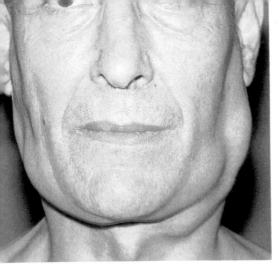

220

220 This man's white cell count is 78 x 10⁹/1 with a differential count of 3% neutrophils and 97% lymphocytes.
  a What is the likely diagnosis?
  b Name three ways in which this condition may give rise to jaundice.
  c What is the immediate effect of prednisolone on the white cell count?

221 a What name is given to this lesion?
      b What treatment is necessary?

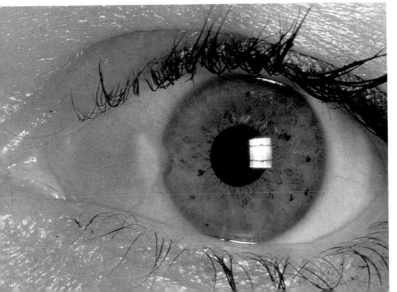

221

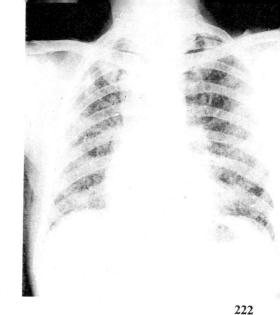

222

222 and 223 This patient complains of non-productive cough of three months duration.

a What principal abnormality is seen on chest x-ray.

b Describe the abnormality seen on skull x-ray?

c What condition is suggested by these appearances?

223

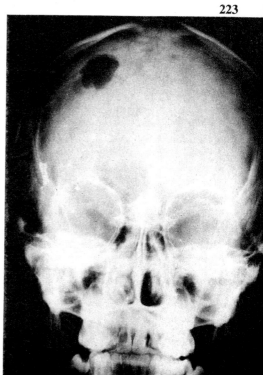

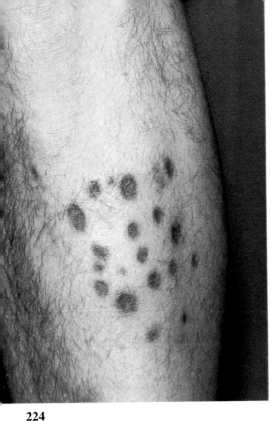

224 This patient is on long-term treatment for a psychotic disorder. He presents with a gradual increase in the number of these lesions on his left shin.
  a What is the most likely cause of these lesions?
  b What is the typical distribution of such lesions?

225 This patient has rheumatoid arthritis.
  a What abnormality is seen at the elbow?
  b What two simple tests are useful in indicating the nature of the swelling?

224

225

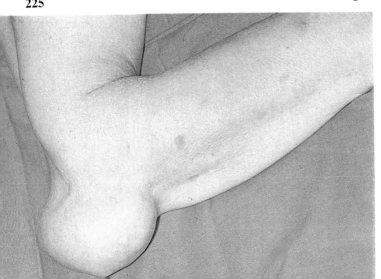

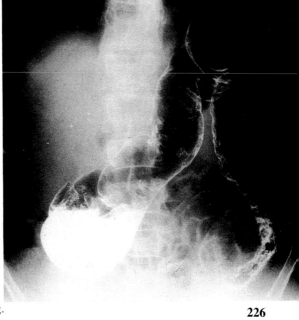

226

227

226 and 227 This patient suffers from recurrent bloody diarrhoea. The lesion seen on her nose began as a tender red nodule, which became bluish before ulcerating. The appearance has changed little over the past four weeks.

a List four abnormal features seen on double contrast barium enema.

b What is the most likely diagnosis?

c What name is given to the skin condition?

d List three other causes of this skin disorder.

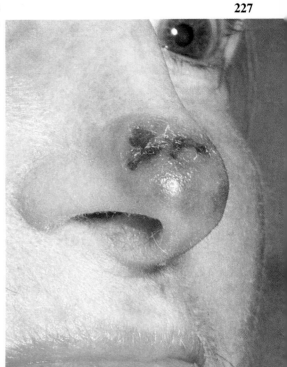

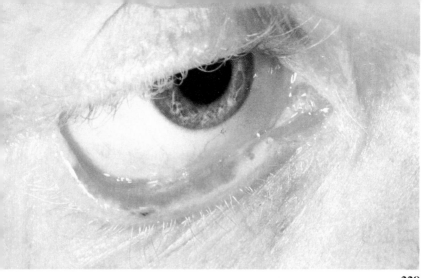

228

228 and 229 This man presented with weight loss, low grade fever and a cardiac murmur. Blood cultures grew streptococcus bovis.
a What is the diagnosis?
b What is the likely source of this organism?
c What is unusual about its antibiotic sensitivity?
d With what condition is this infection associated?

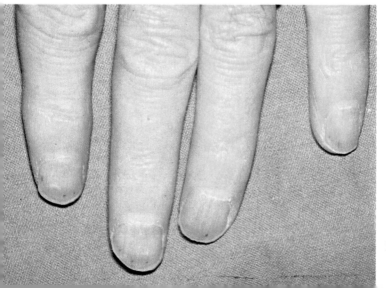

229

230 a What name is given to
this appearance?
  b Which organisms may
be involved?
  c What other condition is
usually present?

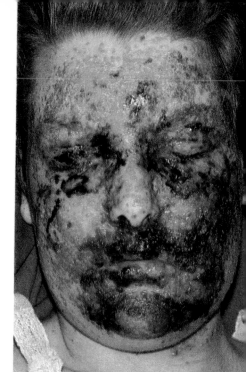

230

231 a Describe the abnormalities present.
  b What is the likely aetiology?
  c What is the most likely predisposing factor in this case?

231

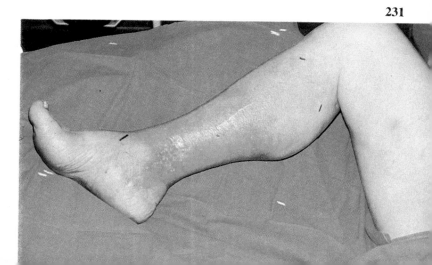

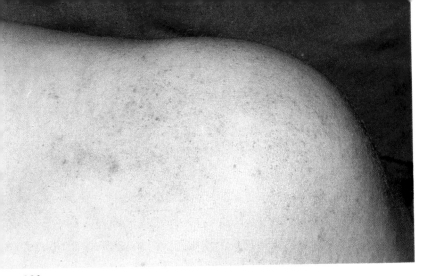

232

223

232 This young patient has become confused and aggressive shortly after his admission to a casualty ward.
What is the cause of his confusion?

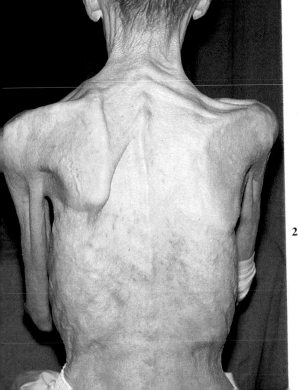

233 This cachectic patient has an intrathoracic neoplasm.
  a What neurological abnormality is shown?
  b Which muscle is affected?
  c In this case, what is the likely underlying cause?

234 This patient complained of recurring inflammation of his ears and nose and occasional 'rheumatic' pains in his chest, accompanied by fever. On several occasions, he had been treated for erysipelas with benzyl penicillin, with no response.
  a What is the diagnosis?
  b How may the diagnosis be established?
  c Which complications may be life-threatening?

235 This immigrant patient complains of recurrent colicky abdominal pain and constipation.
  a What abnormality is shown?
  b What is the diagnosis?
  c Give four other clinical features of this disorder.

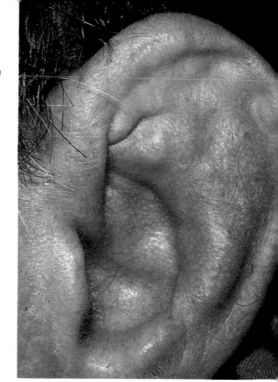

234

235

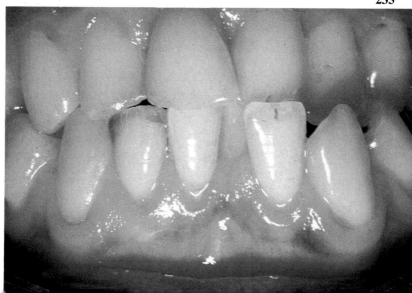

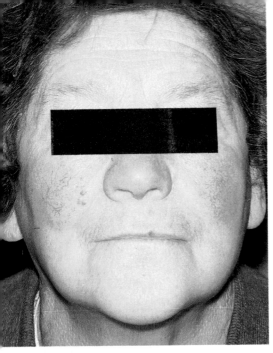

236 This woman presented with tiredness and increasing weight. Laboratory findings included a macrocytic anaemia which showed no improvement following folic acid or vitamin B12 administration.
   a What is the cause of her symptoms?
   b How should her anaemia be treated?

236

237

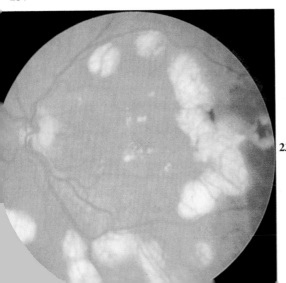

237 This patient is an insulin-dependent diabetic. What are the lesions seen in the periphery of the fundus?

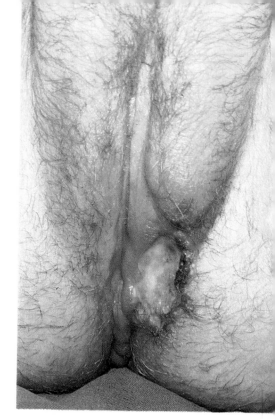

238

238 and 239 This woman presented with recurrent painful ulcers as demonstrated.

a What is the likely diagnosis?

b What other organ is classically involved?

c What laboratory test is diagnostic of this condition?

d Which sex is more likely to be affected?

239

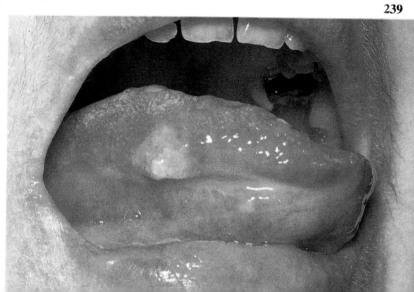

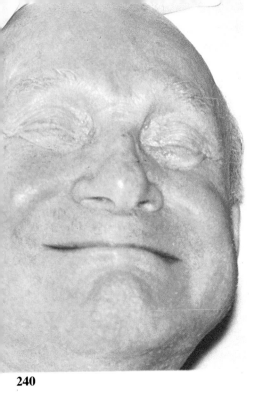

240 This 'smile' is involuntary.
  a What name is given to this appearance?
  b What is its cause?
  c Suggest two drugs which may give rise to a similar appearance

240

241

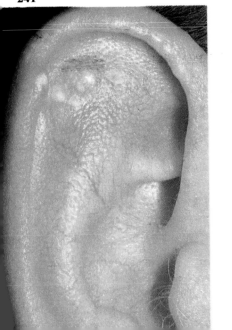

241 This patient suffers from recurrent episodes of joint pain and swelling.
  a What are these lesions?
  b Which two investigations would be most helpful in establishing the diagnosis?

242 This girl presented at the age of eighteen years with primary amenorrhoea and small stature. Neurological examination reveals a bitemporal upper quadrantic visual field defect.

a What is the likely diagnosis?

b Suggest two radiological and three endocrine investigations that should be done.

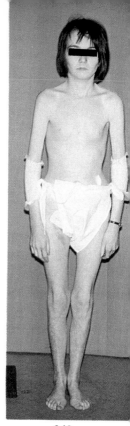

242

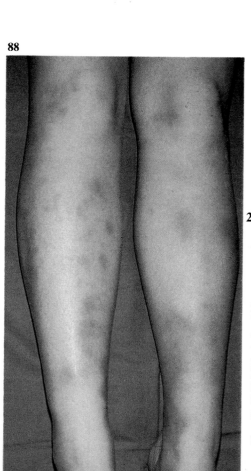

243

243
This twenty-three year old woman presented with a short history of pain and swelling in one knee, fever, and tender lumps over her shins and forearms.

a What are these lesions on her shins?

b Suggest three causes of her illness.

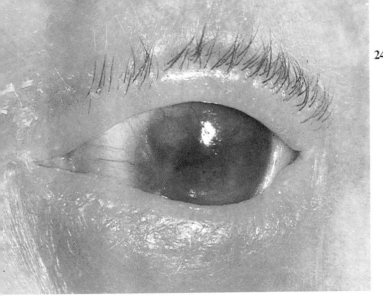

244

244 and 245 This teenage boy complains of pain and loss of vision, initially in the left eye alone, but affecting the right eye a few months later. The abdominal x-ray is that of his mother.

a What is the cause of his visual loss?
b What principal abnormality is seen on the x-ray?
c What is the underlying diagnosis?

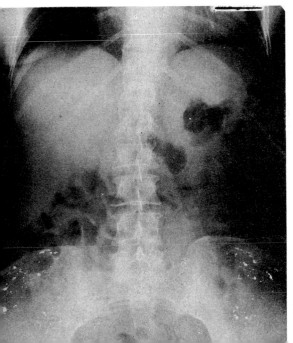

245

246 This patient is of Central African origin.
- a What abnormality is seen in the ocular fundus?
- b What are the two most common infective causes of such an appearance?

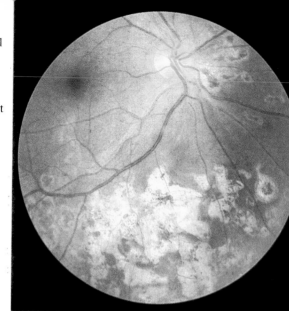

246

247 This patient has scabies.
- a Which variety of this condition gives rise to the appearance seen in this finger web?
- b What is the causative agent?
- c List three conditions which may predispose to this variety.

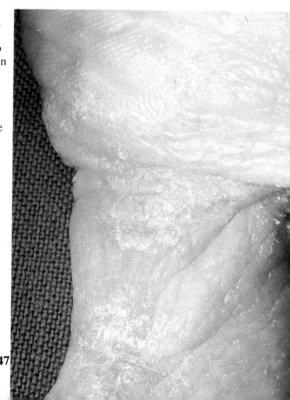

247

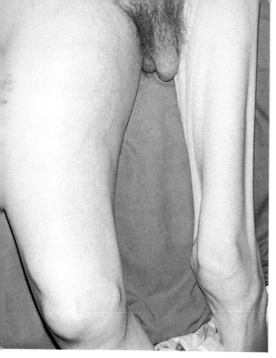

248

249

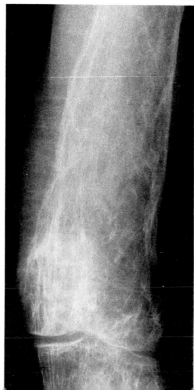

248 and 249 This elderly male patient suffers from a chronic bony disorder. Recently he has complained of pain in the right thigh.

a List four physical abnormalities seen in the legs.

b What radiological abnormalities are visible?

c What is the underlying disorder?

d What is the cause of his pain?

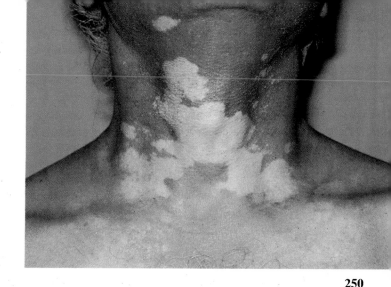

250

250 a What skin lesion is
  shown in this Asian
  patient?
  b What endocrinopathies
  are associated with this
  skin condition?

251

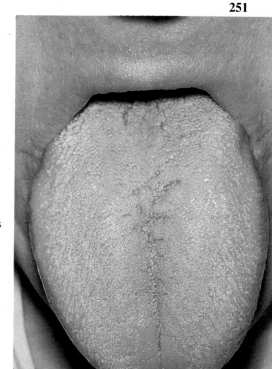

251 This patient is
  hypertensive.
  a What abnormality is
  seen here?
  b What unusual
  underlying cause for his
  hypertension does this
  suggest?

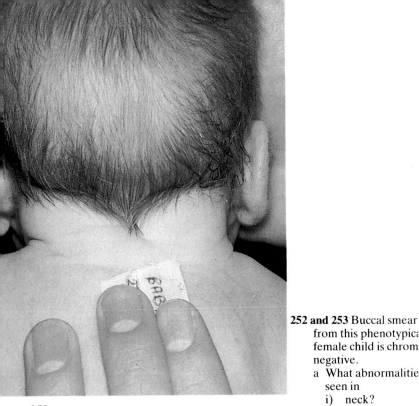

252

252 and 253 Buccal smear from this phenotypically female child is chromatin negative.
  a What abnormalities are seen in
    i) neck?
    ii) feet?
  b What is the likely diagnosis?

253

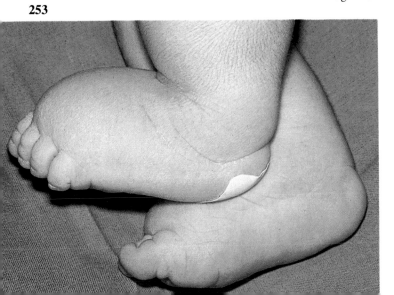

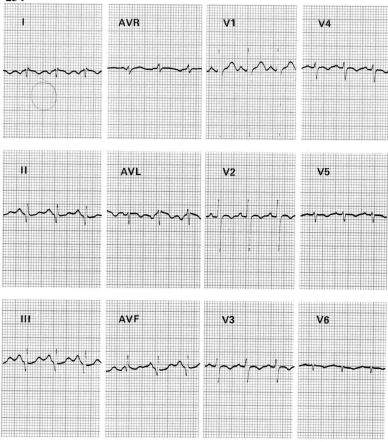

254 This woman with a past history of bronchiectasis was admitted with a further exacerbation. The ECG technician was chastised by the resident medical officer for transposing the limb leads of the ECG.

a Was the resident correct?

b Which diagnosis should be considered?

c What other symptoms may she have?

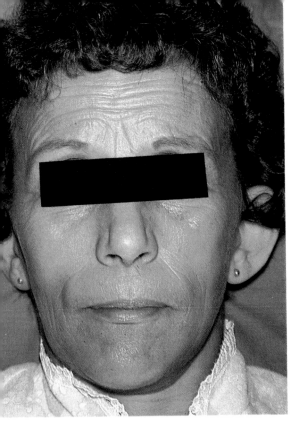

255

This woman has 'bronze diabetes'.

a What is unusual about the diagnosis in this patient?

b What is the cause of the pigmentation?

c What is the mode of inheritance of this disease?

d What is the effect of venesection on
  i) diabetic control?
  ii) cardiac failure?
  iii) risk of hepatoma?

255

256

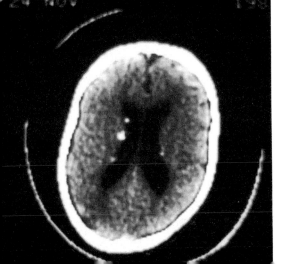

256 This person has epilepsy.

a What abnormality is present in this cerebral CT scan?

b What is the diagnosis?

c What cardiac abnormality is associated with this condition?

257

This person's blood film shows acanthocytosis.
a What abnormality is demonstrated?
b What is the association between these conditions?
c What neurological symptoms may occur?
d What therapy may be helpful in their prevention?

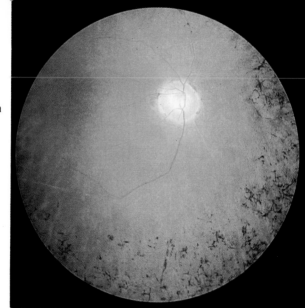

257

258

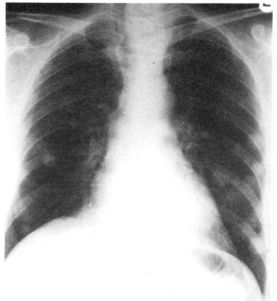

258
a What two abnormalities are seen on this chest x-ray?
b What is the most likely diagnosis?

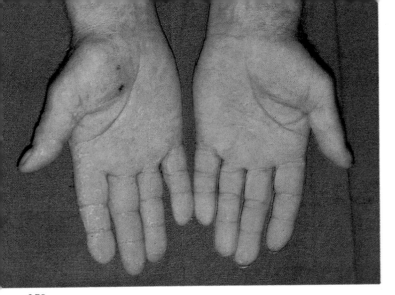

259

260

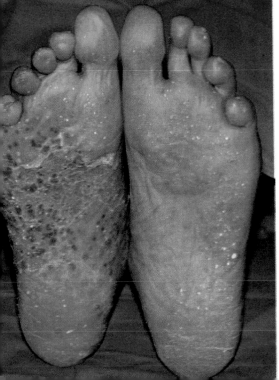

259 and 260 This patient complains of pain and swelling of his knee joints and of painful red eyes. Suggest two diagnoses which link his symptoms with the appearance of his palms and soles.

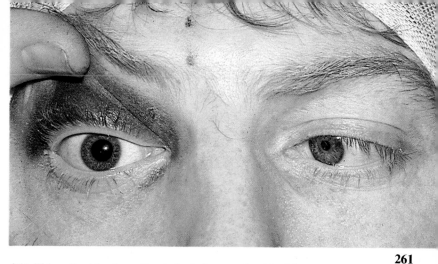

261 This patient is attempting to look down and to his right.
   a What neurological abnormalities are demonstrated?
   b From his appearance, suggest three possible causes.

261

262

262 Which congenital
abnormality is most
typically associated with
this appearance in a
young patient?

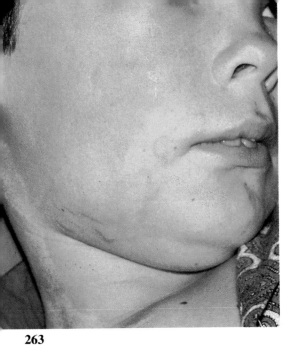

263
What is the cause of this child's recently diagnosed apical diastolic murmur?

263

264

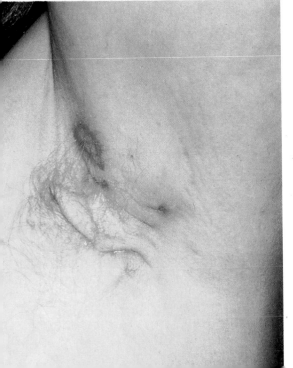

264
a What is the most likely cause of the abnormality seen in this twenty-six year old female patient's axilla?
b Which infective agent is usually responsible?

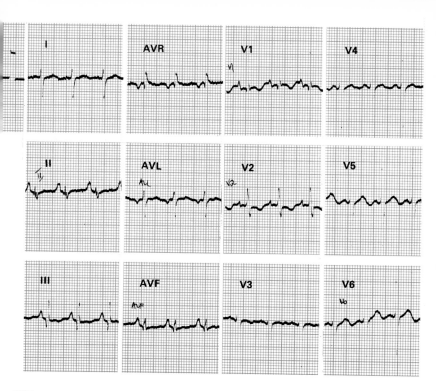

265

265 This thirty-eight year old woman suffers from bronchiectasis following
an attack of measles in childhood.
a What are the ECG abnormalities?
b What condition has developed?

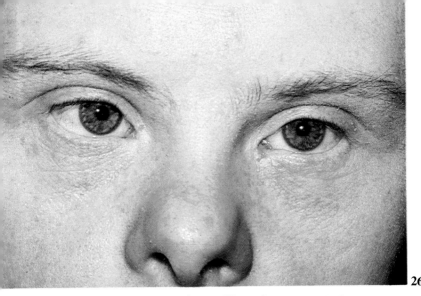

266

266 This patient has Down's syndrome. His mother was twenty-two years old when he was born.
  a List two possible chromosomal abnormalities consistent with this syndrome.
  b List the possible underlying defective genetic mechanisms in order of likelihood.

267 a What abnormality is seen in this lateral skull x-ray?
  b Of what condition is this appearance characteristic?
  c List four other conditions which may give rise to a similar appearance in this area.

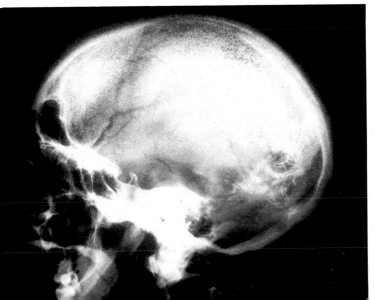

267

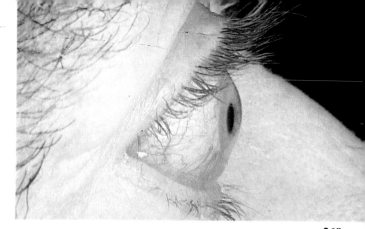

268

269

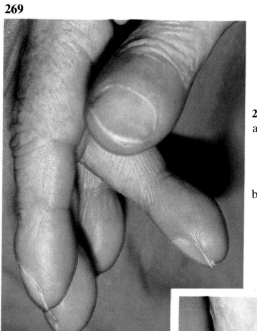

268, 269 and 270

a What abnormalities are
   seen in these patients'
   i)   eye?
   ii) hands?
   iii) legs?
b Which endocrine
   disorder is typified by
   this triad?

270

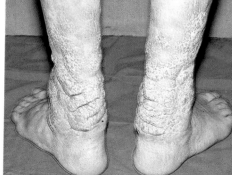

271 a What is this condition?
   b What are the important clinical dermatological features?
   c What is the incidence of systemic lupus erythematosus in this disease?

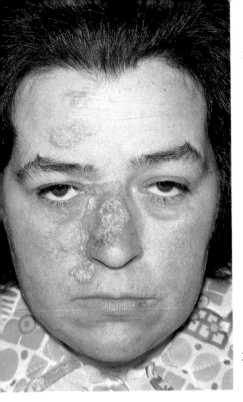

271

272 a What is the cause of the abnormal appearance of this child's eye?
   b What is its aetiology?
   c At which other sites may it be found in the orbit?

272

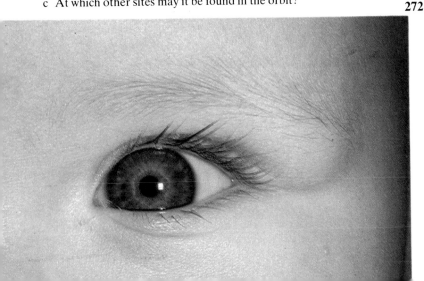

273

This fifty year old man sustained an anterior myocardial infarction. Four days after admission he suddenly became breathless, hypotensive, and peripherally cyanosed. A loud pansystolic murmur was noted.

a What is the radiological diagnosis?

b What is the likely cause of his deterioration?

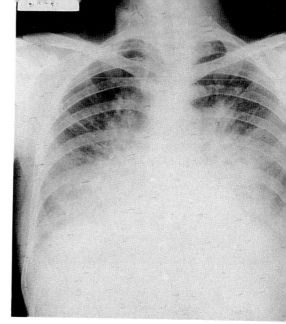

273

274 This man complained of pain on swallowing and pain in his right ear.
  a Describe the abnormality present?
  b What is the likely diagnosis?
  c What factors are involved in its aetiology?

274

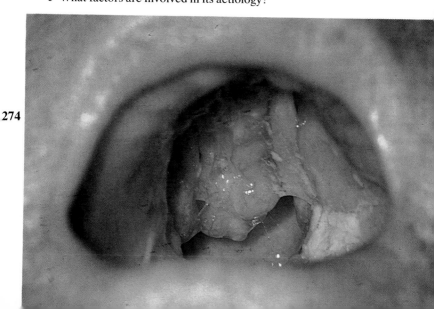

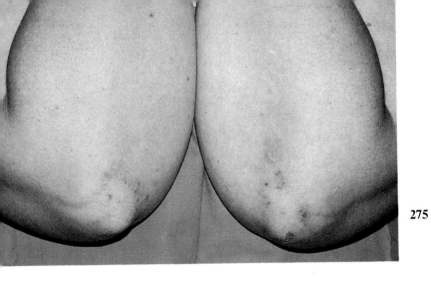

275

275, 276, 277 and 278 These four patients suffer from recurrent
bullous eruptions.
Patient 1
complains of an intensely pruritic eruption on his elbows (as shown),
knees and buttocks. Topical corticosteroid applications have failed to
alleviate the pruritus.
Patient 2
is seventy-five years old. She suffers from recurrent episodes of
blistering of arms, legs and trunk. The blisters are tense, do not rupture
easily, and heal without scarring.

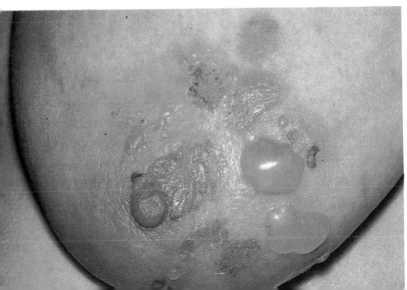

276

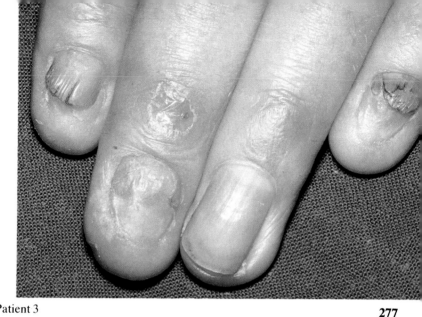

Patient 3
has a strong family history
of blistering disease.
From early childhood,
minor trauma has caused
blistering. The blisters
heal with scarring as
shown.
Patient 4
is fifty-two years old.
Several months ago she
complained of recurrent
painful lesions of the
buccal mucosa. The
blisters seen here are
confined to the left arm.
They are easily broken,
leaving painful, raw areas
beneath.
Give the most likely
diagnosis in each case.

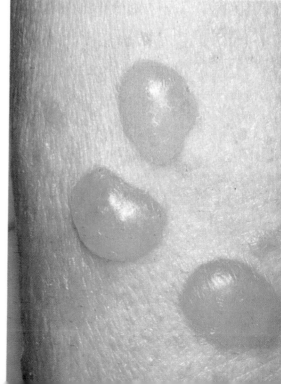

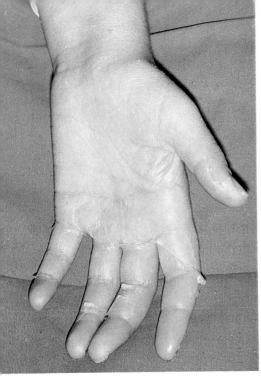

279 and 280 These conditions have an aetiological link.
  a What are the conditions?
  b What is the link?
  c What accounts for the differing clinical presentation?

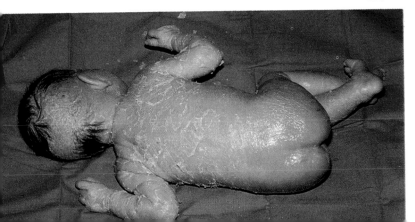

281

This patient is attempting to smile.
a What is the diagnosis?
b By which investigation is this most easily established?
c What other investigations are useful?

281

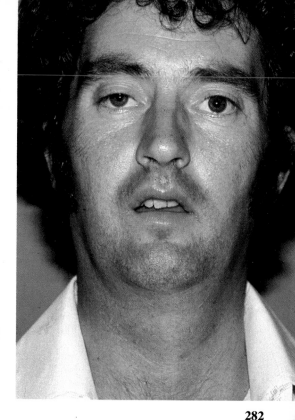

282

282

This patient has a recent history of pain in the tongue and jaw on chewing. Twelve hours ago she suddenly became blind in this eye.
a List three abnormalities visible in the optic fundus.
b What is the diagnosis?
c Would you expect the indirect light reflex in this eye to be normal?
d What underlying diagnosis must be considered?

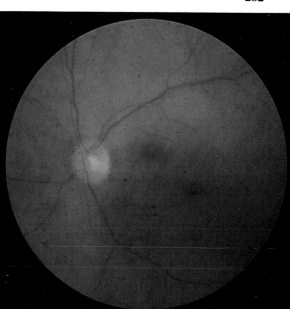

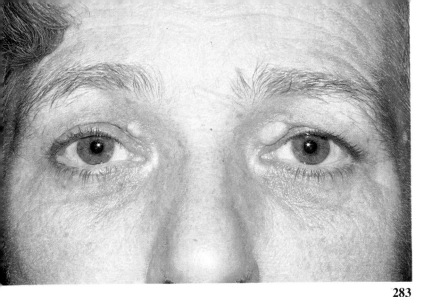

283

283 and 284 This thirty-six year old woman has a strong family history of ischaemic heart disease.
  a What abnormality is seen adjacent to her eyelids?
  b What substance is responsible for the yellow discolouration of her hands?
  c Suggest five conditions which may be associated with both abnormalities.

284

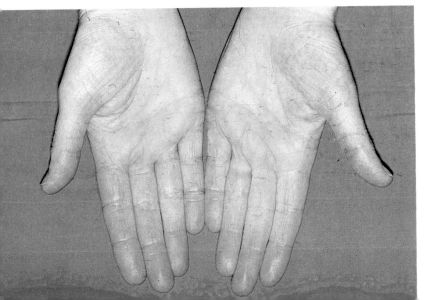

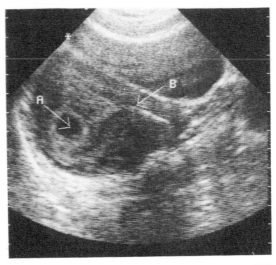

285

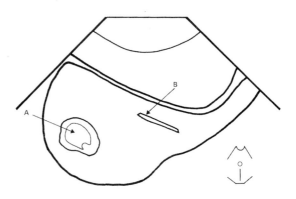

285 This nineteen year old girl presented with back pain in the lower lumbar area. A pelvic mass was found on examination and a diagnosis of ovarian cyst was made.
a Does this sagittal ultrasonic pelvic scan confirm this diagnosis?
b Name the features labelled 'A' and 'B'.

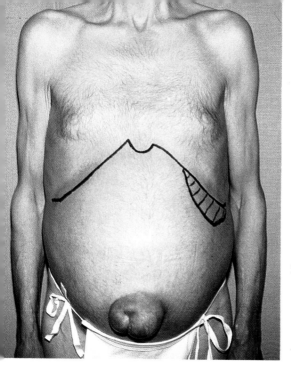

286 This patient has ascites.

a In addition to splenomegaly (delineated in pen) which two other principal abnormalities are visible?

b What is, approximately, the smallest amount of ascitic fluid which can be detected clinically? By which unusual test may this be detected?

287 This patient works in a glue factory. The lesion seen on her left cheek began as a small scratch a week ago. Over the past four days the lesion has enlarged rapidly. She now complains of headache and malaise. Her temperature is 38°C and pulse rate 90/minute.

a What other facial abnormality is seen?

286

287

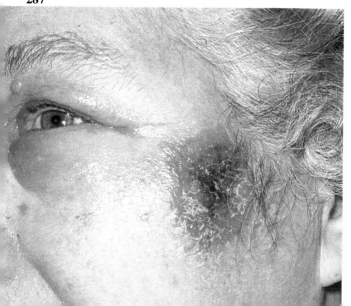

b Of which unusual infection is this appearance typical?
c What other conditions may give rise to a similar appearance?
d Is specific treatment necessary?

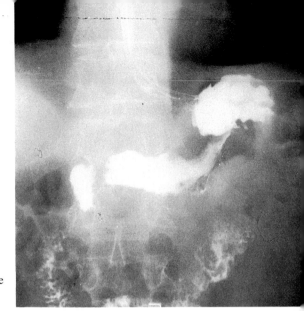

88 This fifty year old male patient complains of weight loss and fullness after meals.
  a What abnormality is seen on barium meal?
  b What descriptive name is given to this lesion?

288

289

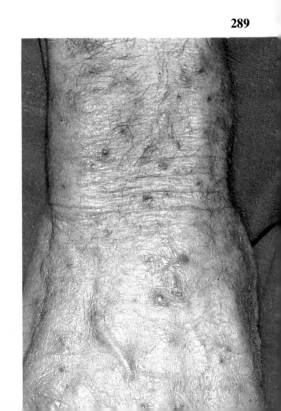

289 This patient has an iron deficiency anaemia. Faecal occult blood analysis is consistently positive. Gastroscopy, sigmoidoscopy and barium series have demonstrated no abnormalities.
  a What unusual diagnosis is suggested by the appearance of the skin of his forearm?
  b What is the source of blood loss in this condition?
  c In which other sites may similar lesions occur?

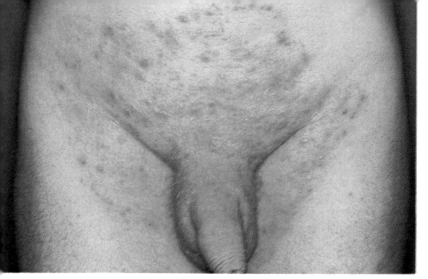

290

291

290 This man's itchy rash
flared up when he applied
a topical steroid cream.
a What is the likely
underlying aetiology?
b What therapy should
he have been
prescribed?

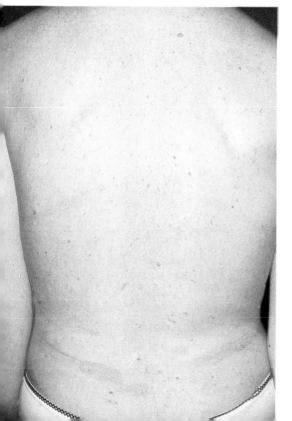

291
This thirty-three year old
woman presented with
left sensorineural
deafness and tinnitus of
three month's duration.
Examination revealed an
absent left corneal reflex.
a What two skin
abnormalities are seen?
b What is the underlying
disorder?
c What is the cause of her
deafness?

292 This boy with choreoathetosis and a tendency to self mutilation has had several episodes of gout.
  a What is the name of this condition?
  b How is it inherited?
  c Which enzyme is lacking?

293 This obese female patient has been admitted following a haematemesis.
  a What name is given to the venous abnormality seen in relation to her umbilicus?
  b What underlying haemodynamic disturbance does this imply?
  Which three causes for her haematemesis should be considered?

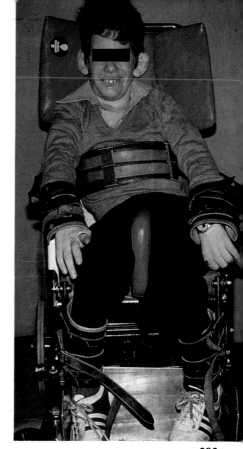

292

293

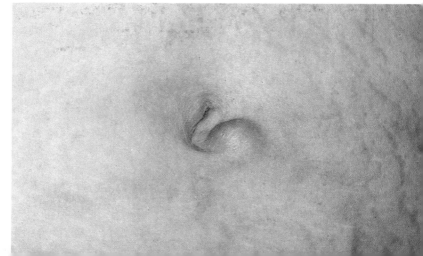

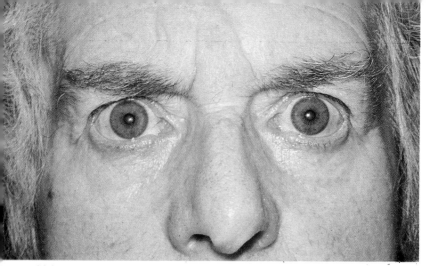

294

294 and 295
    a What physical sign is being demonstrated here?
    b What is the significance of a positive test?

295

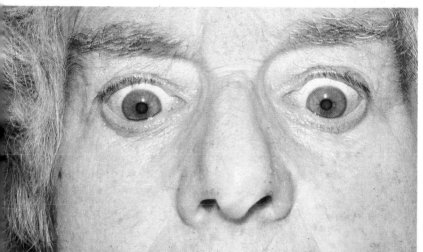

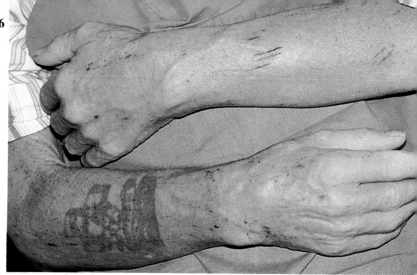

296

296 and 297 This patient has been admitted to your unit moribund and unable to give a history. He is hypotensive and clinically dehydrated, tachypnoeic with Kussmaul-type respiration. His previous case notes are not available, but you are able to locate his previous x-rays. Initial biochemical results are: Na 148 mmol/l, K 6.2 mmol/l, HCO_3 7 mmol/l, urea 42.0 mmol/l, creatinine 440 mol/l, plasma glucose 5.8 mmol/l.

a What abnormalties are seen
  i)   in the hand x-rays?
  ii) on the skin of his arms?
b What important implication can be taken, with respect to his pre-existing renal function?
c What value, approximately, would you expect the urinary specific gravity to be?

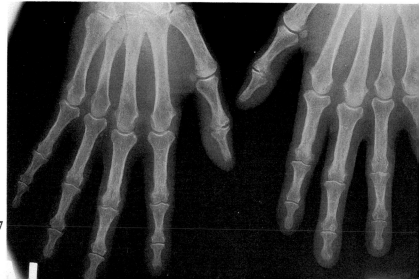

297

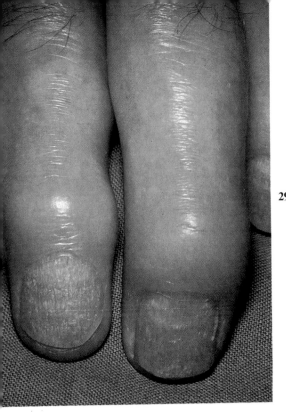

298

298 and 299 This patient complained of morning stiffness and pain in the small joints of the hand. A diagnosis of rheumatoid arthritis was made. After six months on a variety of nonsteroidal anti-inflammatory drugs he was given a 'second line' drug. Shortly afterwards he developed widespread erythroderma with pustulation.

a What was the true cause of his joint pains?

b Which 'second line' drug was he given?

299

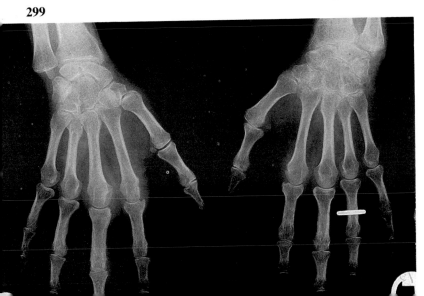

300

a What principal
  abnormality is seen on
  this chest radiograph?
b What is the diagnosis?
c In which two other sites
  would you expect to
  find radiological
  abnormalities in this
  condition?

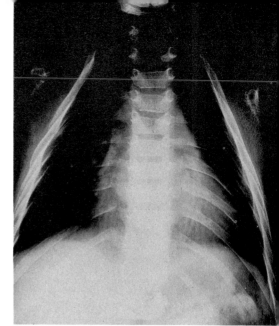

300

301

301

a What physical sign is
  demonstrated here?
b What is the significance
  of this finding?

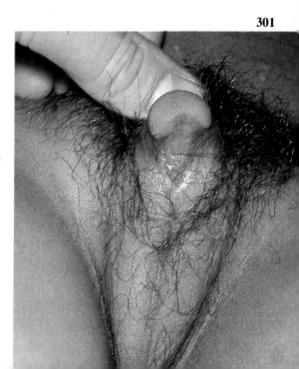

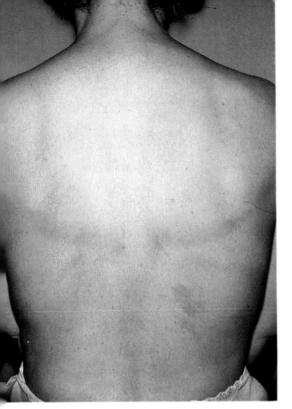

302

This woman presented
with a six month history
of general ill-health,
weight loss of two stones,
and light headedness.

a What diagnosis does
   her appearance
   suggest?
b How should the
   diagnosis be
   confirmed?
c What abnormalities
   may a differential white
   cell count show?

302

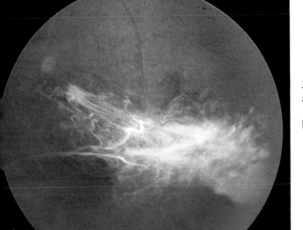

303

a What is this
   appearance?
b In which diseases may
   it occur?

303

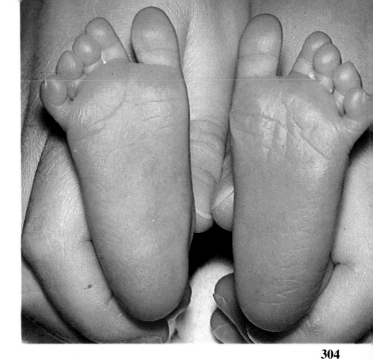

304

304 Is this a full term baby?

305 a What is the cause of this appearance?
   b What effect on function occurs?
   c What iatrogenic factor may be involved?

305

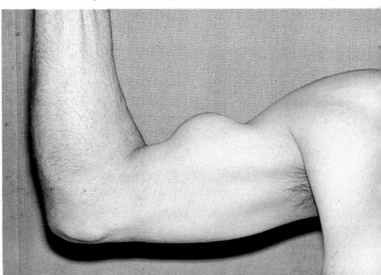

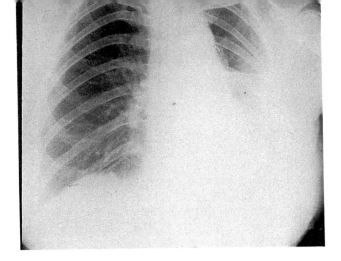

306

306 and 307 These x-rays were taken three years apart, the lower most
recently.
   a List four radiological abnormalities visible in the upper x-ray.
   b What new abnormality has developed in the lower x-ray?
   c What is the likely diagnosis?

307

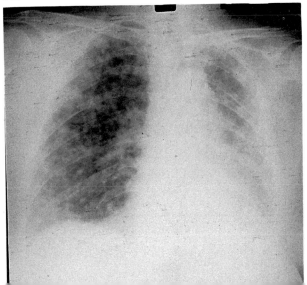

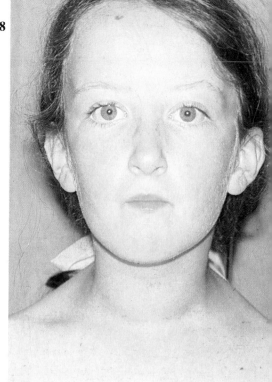

308 This girl is clinically mildly hyperthyroid. Her total serum thyroxine (T4) concentration is at the upper limit of normal at 148 nmol/l. She has received neither antithyroid nor ablative therapy. Suggest five possible reasons for the apparently low T4.

309 This seventy year old lady was admitted with acute abdominal pain radiating through to her back. The pain was accompanied by abdominal tenderness.
Name the structures labelled 1 to 5 on this CT scan of the lower abdomen (following intravenous injection of contrast medium).

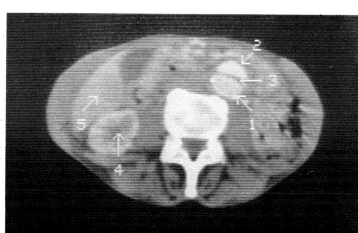

309

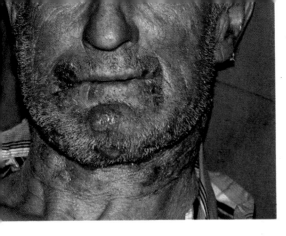

310 This farmer blamed his cows for his facial appearance.
    a Is he correct?
    b What is the diagnosis?
    c What treatment is indicated?

311 Name four organisms which may cause this appearance.

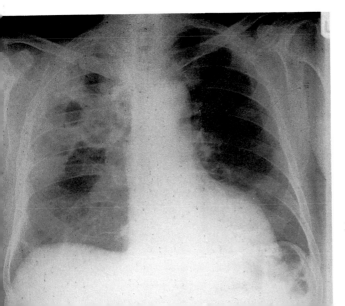

312

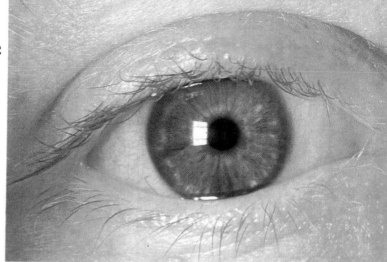

312 This patient is a fish-filleter. She developed severe headache and myalgia, followed by sore eyes. On admission, she was jaundiced, had calf pain and microscopic haematuria.
   a What is the likely diagnosis?
   b Is her occupation relevant?
   c What is the major vector of the disease?

313 This child developed an itchy papule on the dorsum of his hand which has continued to spread.
   a What is the diagnosis?
   b Which agent is usually responsible?

313

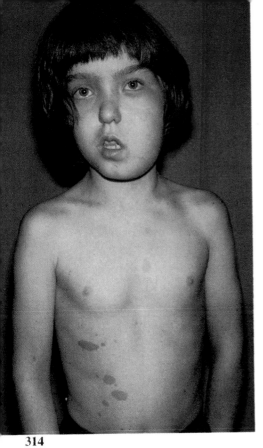

314 This child's facial nerve palsy has an unusual underlying cause. Suggest what this cause may be.

315 This patient complains of severe unremitting headache, excessive sweating and pins and needles in his hands and forearms.
  a What diagnosis is suggested by the radiological appearance of his hands?
  b What is the likely cause of his paraesthesiae?

314

315

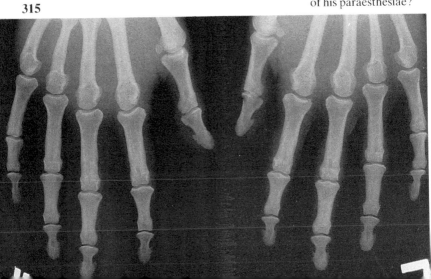

316

This twenty year old patient has a refractory error.

a What name is given to the abnormal fundal appearance?

b Is the eyeball likely to be abnormally long or abnormally short?

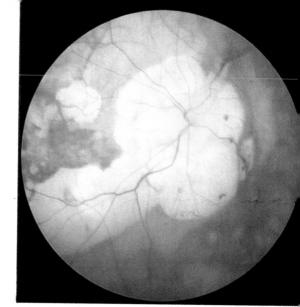

316

317

317

This patient has recently been aware of flu-like symptoms. Two weeks ago she developed a generalised rash. She has generalised lymphadenopathy and her blood pressure is 190/120. Urine microscopy reveals red cells and red cell casts.

a What is the underlying diagnosis?

b What abnormality would you expect on renal biopsy?

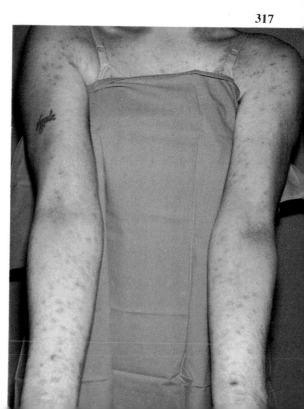

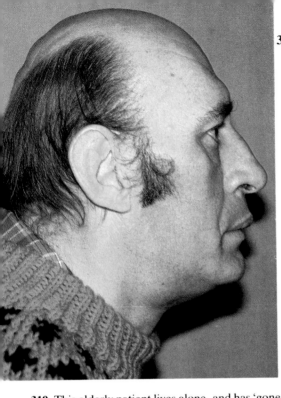

318

318 This man is acromegalic. Name five abnormalities which may be seen on a lateral skull x-ray.

319 This elderly patient lives alone, and has 'gone off her legs'. There is no history of fall, other injury or clinical evidence of a haemorrhagic diathesis. She has a normochromic anaemia, with normal white cell and platelet counts. The Hess test is positive.
a What is the likely cause of the bruising seen here?
b She is edentulous. Would you expect to find evidence of the above condition in her gums?
c How is the diagnosis established biochemically?

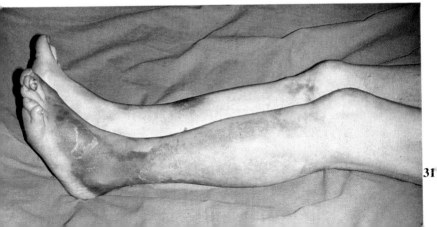

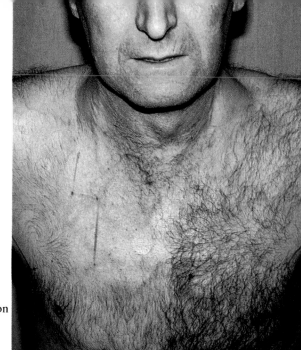

320

320 and 321

This patient complains of headache on awakening in the morning, of one week's duration.

a What abnormalities are seen on
   i) his chest wall?
   ii) his chest x-ray?
b What is the cause of his symptoms and what is the most likely diagnosis?
c What treatment has he received?

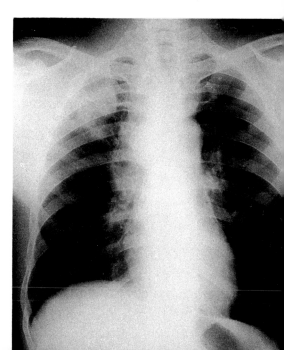

321

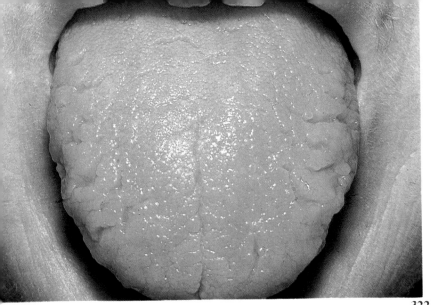

322 This woman experiences recurrent swelling of her lips.
 a What abnormality is shown?
 b What else is she likely to suffer from?
 c What is this condition called?

322

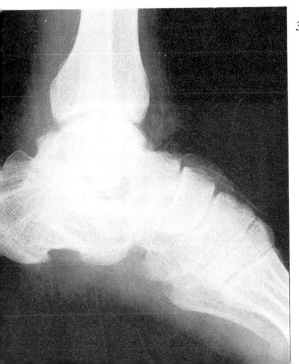

323

323
This diabetic patient has severe peripheral vascular disease. Following minor trauma to a toenail, he has experienced increasingly severe pain in the forefoot.
 a What radiological abnormality is visible?
 b What is the diagnosis?

324 This patient's sclerae are white. Recently he has complained of increased swelling of the lower right tibia, with intense pain locally.
  a What is the underlying diagnosis?
  b What complication has developed?

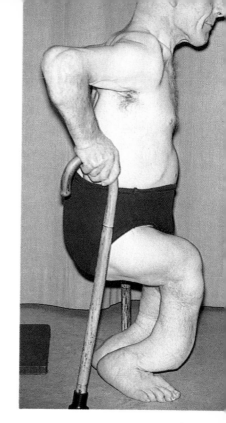

324

325 This woman has normal vision.
  a What is this lesion?
  b What treatment is indicated?

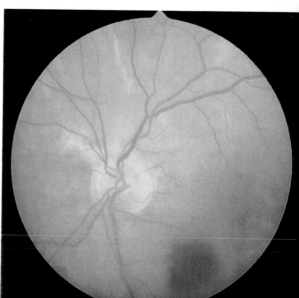

325

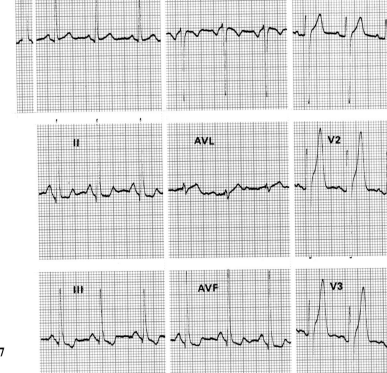

326 This lesion developed during an exacerbation of chronic obstructive airways disease. It has also appeared during earlier exacerbations, but has always healed, leaving only minimal pigmentation.

a What is the diagnosis?

b What are the two most likely causes in this patient?

c How would you establish the diagnosis?

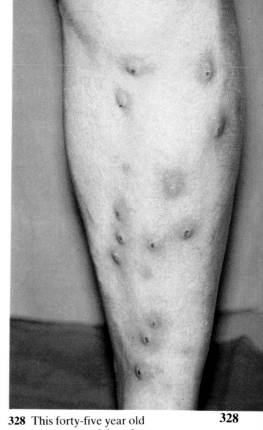

328

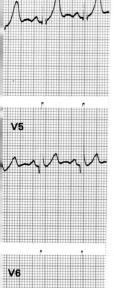

V4

V5

V6

328 This forty-five year old woman complains of intense pruritus of both shins. She dates the symptoms from a visit to her local cinema two years ago.

a What is the diagnosis?

b What form of therapy is usually successful?

327 This is the ECG of a thirty year old man admitted for investigation of dyspepsia.
What immediate action should be taken?

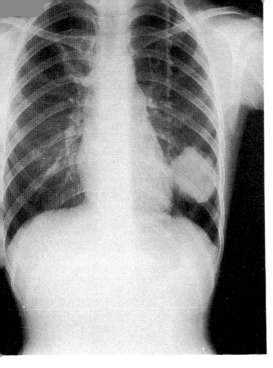

329 This shepherd suffers
from a disease which has
been eradicated from
Iceland.
a What is the diagnosis?
b What is the distribution
of this disease
throughout the world?
c What is man's rôle in
the life-cycle of this
disease?

329

330 a What is this condition?
b Which three groups of
drugs are commonly
responsible for its
development?

330

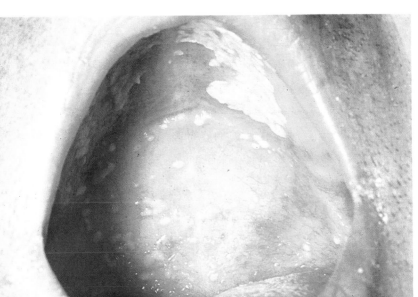

331 a What investigation is
this?
b What abnormality is
present?
c What neurological
abnormalities are
typical of this
condition?

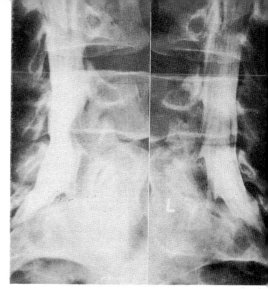

331

332

332 a What is the most likely
cause of the lesion seen
behind this patient's
ear?
b Would you expect to
find submandibular
lymphadenopathy?

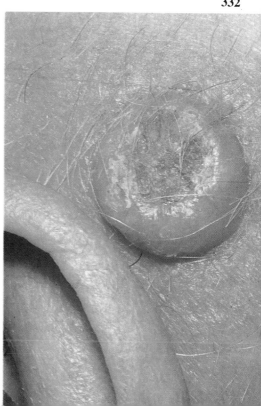

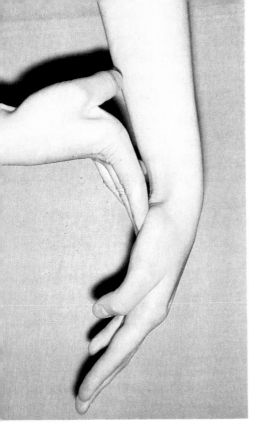

333

333 and 334 This patient has been found to have an apical midsystolic murmur on routine clinical examination.
  a What abnormalities are seen of
  i) the forearms?
  ii) the skin?
  b What is the diagnosis?
  c Which cardiac valvular abnormality, associated with this condition, explains the murmur?

334

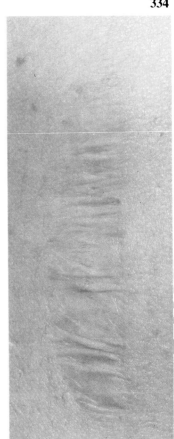

335 This woman is free of symptoms and is on no regular medication.
a What is the most likely cause of her skin pigmentation?
b In what other sites would you expect to find pigmentation in this condition?

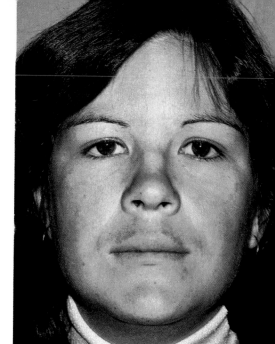

335

336 This patient had an appendicectomy two years ago. She now complains of general malaise of indeterminate onset.
a What abnormality of the appendicectomy scar can be seen?
b What diagnosis does this suggest?
c What information does the scar give about onset of this disorder?

336

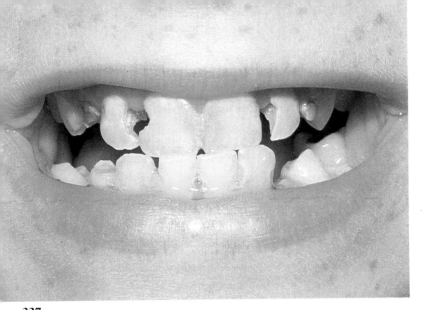

337

338

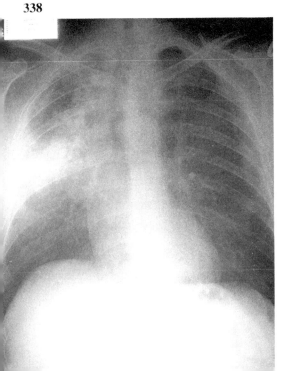

337 and 338 This young man presented with chronic cough, purulent sputum and weight loss. Examination of sputum revealed the presence of sulphur granules.
a What is the diagnosis?
b Which serological test is useful in confirming the diagnosis?
c What is the significance of his dental hygiene?

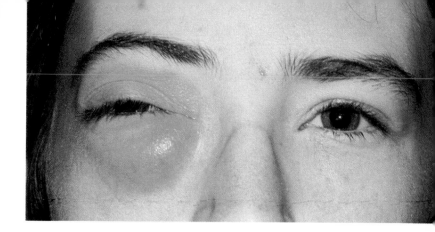

339 a What is this condition?

    b What complications may develop?

    c What signs would indicate involvement of the globe?

340 This woman complained of severe pain in her left forearm and hand for three days. She then developed this vesicular, crusted eruption.

    a What is the diagnosis?

    b Which nerve roots are affected?

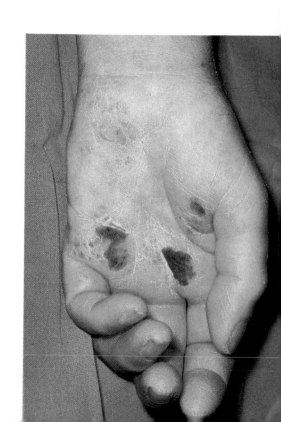

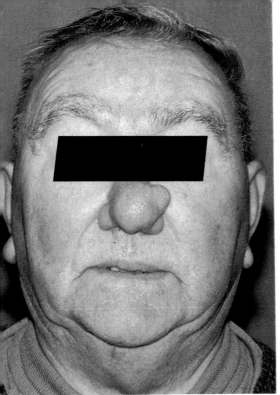

341

341 a What is the most likely
cause of this patient's
facial rash?
 b List four ocular
complications of this
disorder.

342

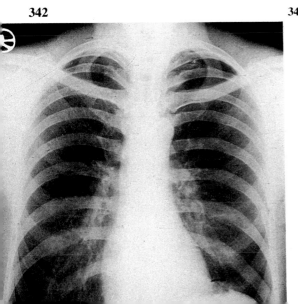

342 This young patient
presents with sudden
onset of pleuritic chest
pain and breathlessness.
  What abnormality is
seen on chest x-ray?

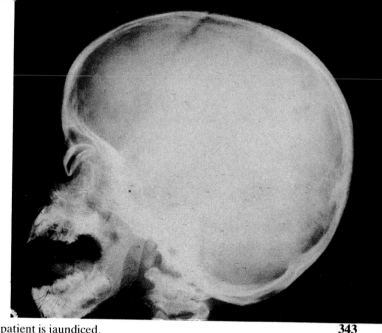

343 This patient is jaundiced.
  a What abnormality is
    seen in the lateral skull
    x-ray?
  b How does this explain
    his jaundice?

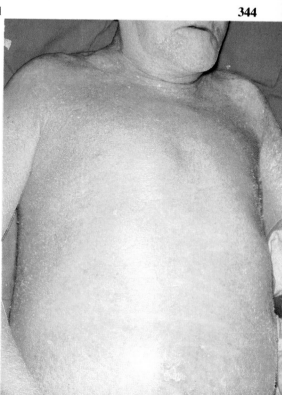

344 This patient complains of
    generalised intense
    pruritus. In addition to
    the skin abnormality, he
    has generalised
    lymphadenopathy. He is
    taking no drugs and there
    is no history of previous
    skin disorder.
  a What dermatological
    abnormality is seen?
  b What underlying
    systemic diseases
    should be considered?
  c List four complications
    of the skin disorder.

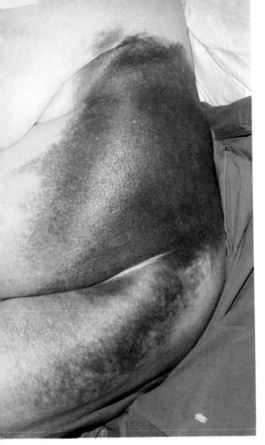

345 This woman has a family history of bleeding and a lifelong personal history of recurrent epistaxis and menorrhagia.
a What is the likely diagnosis?
b What will the bleeding time show?
c What will the result be of platelet aggregation studies with collagen?
d What percentage of her children will be affected?

346 This Indian patient presented with painless swelling of his foot, with multiple draining sinuses from which black granules are occasionally discharged.
a What is the name of this condition?
b Which antibacterial agent is usually successful?
c To which organs does systemic spread occur?

345

346

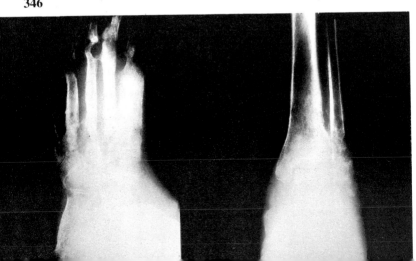

347

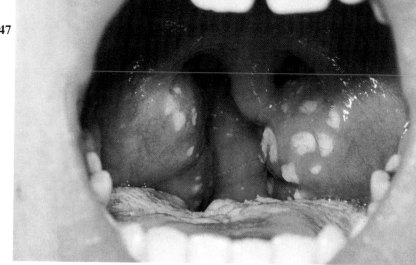

347 What signs will differentiate streptococci from viruses as a cause of this appearance?

348

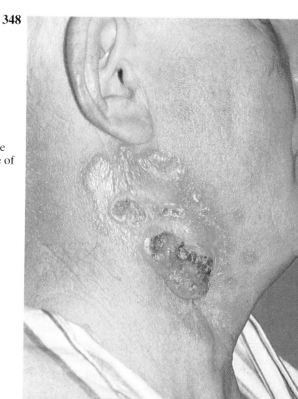

348 This condition was once the healing prerogative of kings.
  a What is its name?
  b Which organism is usually responsible?

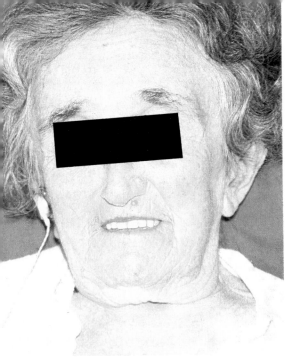

349

349 and 350
 a What is the cause of this patient's deafness?
 b Is specific treatment indicated?

350

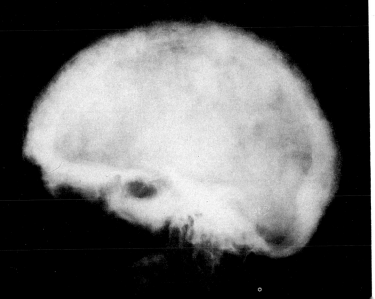

351 This patient has
rheumatoid arthritis.
  a What are these lesions
    seen near the elbow?
  b What are the typical
    histological features of
    such lesions?
  c With which serological
    abnormality are they
    associated?

352 This patient has raised
levels of blood pressure.
  a What anatomical
    abnormality is shown?
  b What diagnosis does
    this suggest?
  c What should be
    considered as a possible
    cause for her raised
    blood pressure?

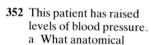

351

352

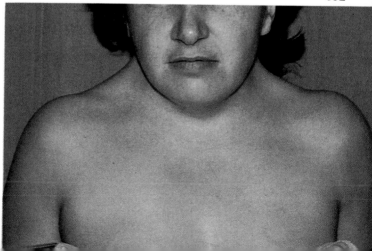

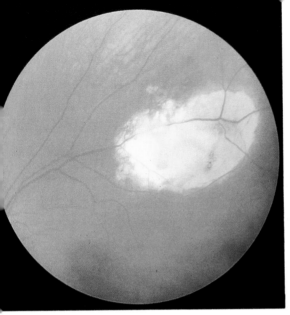

353

353 and 354

a What abnormality is shown in the
   i)   fundus?
   ii) x-ray?
b How may they be associated?

354

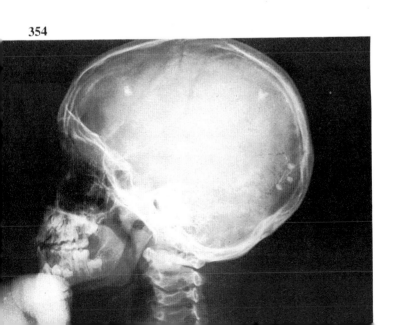

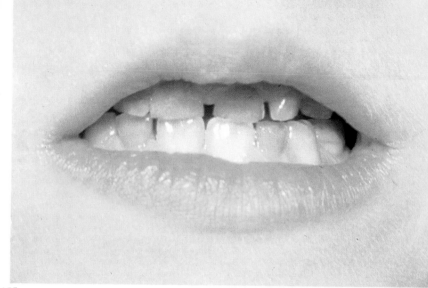

355

355

a What dental abnormality is present and what is the likely cause?

b How can this diagnosis be confirmed clinically?

c What is the cause of the irregularity of the appearance?

d Are these teeth more prone to caries than usual?

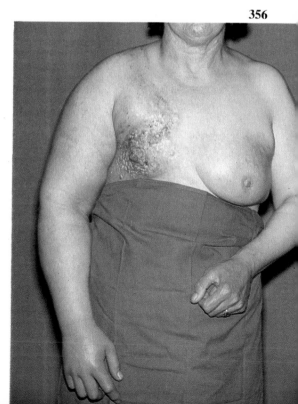

356

This woman received radiotherapy following breast surgery.

a What four abnormalities are present?

b To which rare vascular tumour may this appearance predispose?

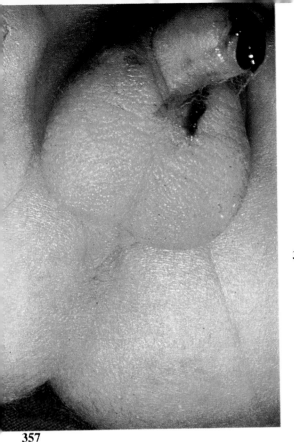

357

357 a What two abnormalities are present?
   b What does this indicate?

359 a What is this condition
   b What underlying diagnosis should you suspect?

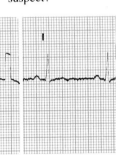

358 This middle aged man suddenly developed paralysis of his left face, arm and leg without disturbance of consciousness. Five days previously he had experienced anterior chest discomfort. Computerised tomography showed a large cerebral infarction in the territory of the right middle cerebral artery. An ECG recorded three months previously was normal.

a What is the likely cause of his stroke?
b Is immediate anticoagulation indicated?
c How might the cause of his stroke be established?

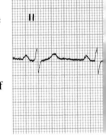

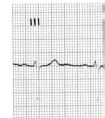

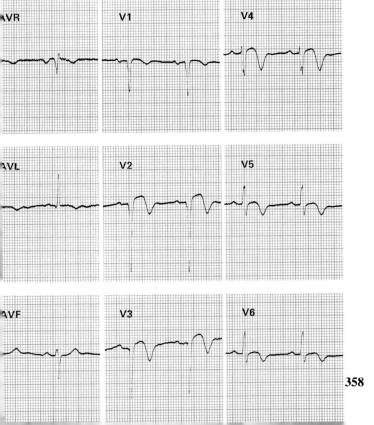

359

358

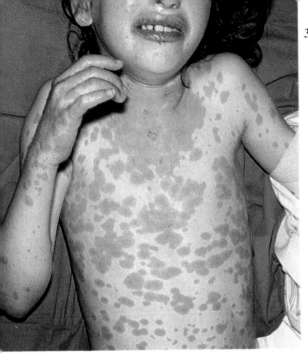

360 and 361
   a What name is given to this girl's rash?
   b Which organisms are most commonly associated with this condition?
   c Are immunofluorescence studies useful in confirming the diagnosis?

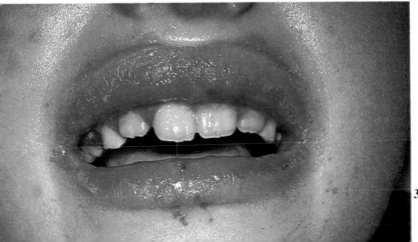

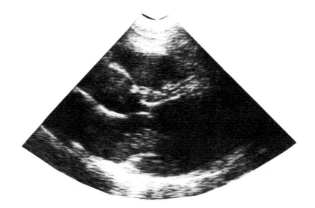

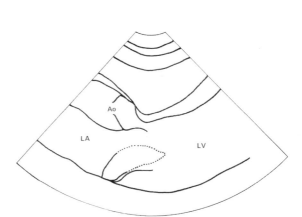

362 This forty-five year old patient presented with a two month history of malaise, weight loss and intermittent fever. There was no history of rheumatic fever in childhood. Auscultation of the heart revealed a third heart sound, with a variable relationship to the second sound and an apical pansystolic murmur. Chest x-ray showed left atrial prominence but no ventricular hypertrophy. Shortly after admission to hospital, she developed transient weakness of the right arm and leg.

   a What abnormality is seen in this cross-sectional echocardiogram through the long axis of the left ventricle?

   b What is the likely diagnosis?

   c What treatment is necessary?

363 This patient, a chronic asthmatic, on regular corticosteroid treatment, has been admitted to an acute medical receiving unit. The appearance shown developed shortly after admission. What is the most likely cause of the appearance of her left groin?

364 This patient, a non-smoker, gives a six month history of night sweats and weight loss. Ten days ago she began to be aware of increasingly severe headache, worse on wakening. Her serum albumin is 35 g/l.

a What abnormality is seen?

b What is the diagnosis?

c What is the most likely underlying pathology?

d What principal abnormality would you expect to see on chest x-ray?

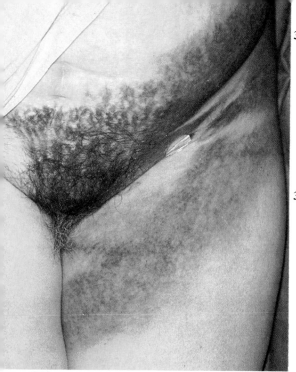

363

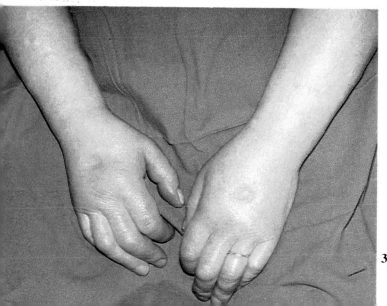

364

365

This patient complains of altered sensation in her feet, "as if walking on cotton wool".

a What two abnormalities are seen?

b What single agent may be responsible?

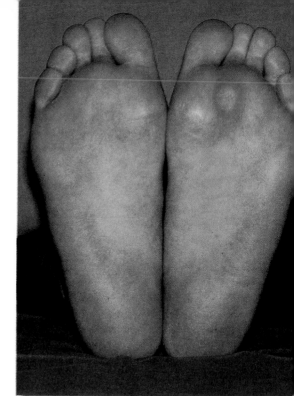

365

366

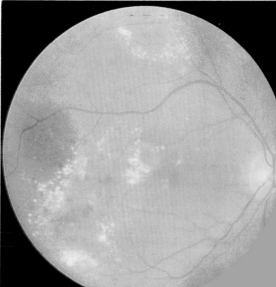

366

a What abnormalities are seen in this optic fundus?

b What investigations would you carry out to diagnose the underlying condition?

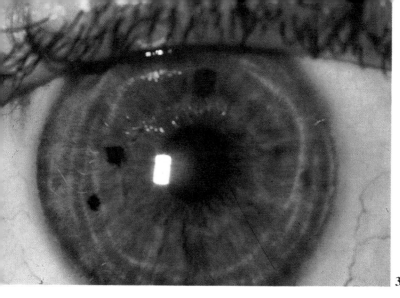

367

367 and 368 This patient has chronic renal failure. His corrected serum calcium is 3.2 mmol/l.
   a What ocular abnormality is seen?
   b What abnormality (apart from the acneiform rash and adhesive plaster) is seen in the picture of his chest?
   c What is the likely endocrine abnormality?

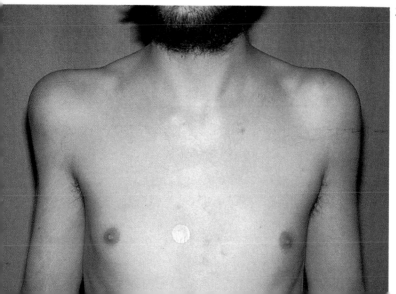

368

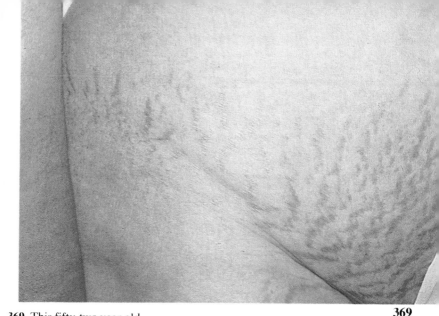

369

369 This fifty-two year old
female patient is
hypertensive.
  a What abnormality is
    seen on the skin of her
    abdomen and thigh?
  b Which underlying
    endocrine disorder
    should be considered?
  c Similar skin changes
    may be seen in normal
    pregnancy. In what way
    do these differ in
    appearance from those
    seen in the above
    condition?

370

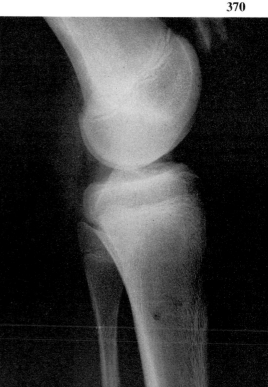

370 This eleven year old boy
presented with pain and
swelling around his
anterior tibial tubercle.
  a What radiological
    abnormality is present?
  b What is the diagnosis?
  c What treatment is
    required?

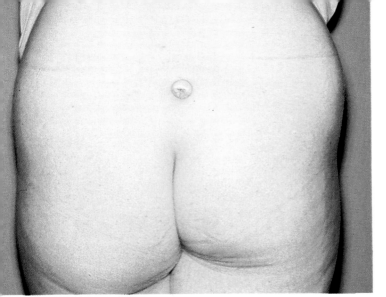

371

372

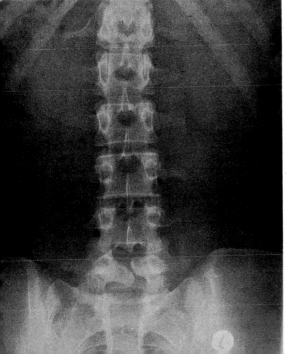

371 and 372 This teenage girl
complains of occasional
urinary incontinence, of
recent onset. She has
bilateral pes cavus and
absent ankle jerks but the
legs are otherwise
neurologically intact.
a What is this condition?
b How does this explain
  her incontinence and
  absent ankle jerks?

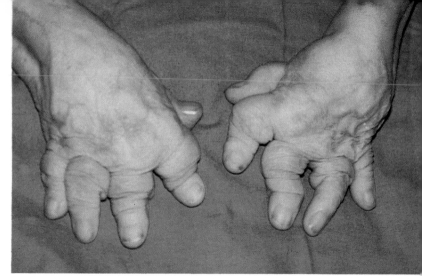

373

373 and 374 Both these patients have severe longstanding joint disease.
  a What descriptive name is given to the degree of joint abnormality
     seen in the hands?
  b Of which condition are these appearances characteristic?
  c What are the three earliest radiological abnormalities in this
     condition?

374

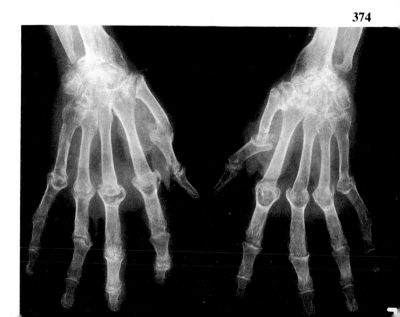

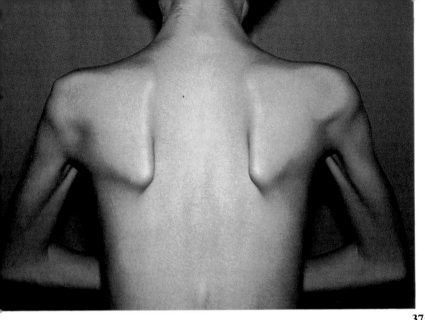

375, 376, 377 and 378 These patients suffer from the same
progressive disorder. The first patient (whose face and back are seen) is
unable to do 'press-ups' at school and cannot whistle, nor use a drinking
straw. He has been asked to bare his teeth. The second patient has, in
addition to severe weakness of the shoulder girdle, a high stepping gait.
The third patient finds that his golf handicap is gradually increasing, but
has no other complaints.

376

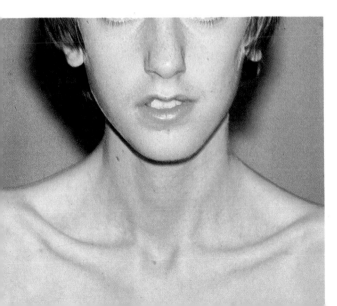

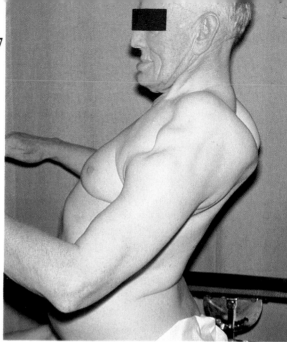

a What is the most likely diagnosis?
b i)   What is the likely cause of the second patient's abnormal gait?
   ii)   What would you expect to find on testing his tendon reflexes?
c Which muscles are most obviously affected in
   i)   the first patient?
   ii) the third patient?
d What effect does this disorder have on life expectancy?

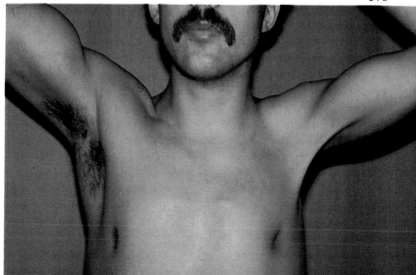

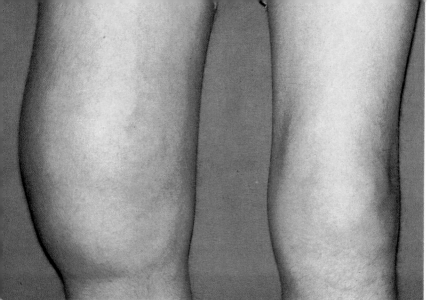

379

379 This teenage patient presents with an acutely swollen and painful knee after a friendly game of football.

  a Why might he be at risk of developing the acquired immune deficiency syndrome?

  b Which other groups are said to be at higher than normal risk?

380

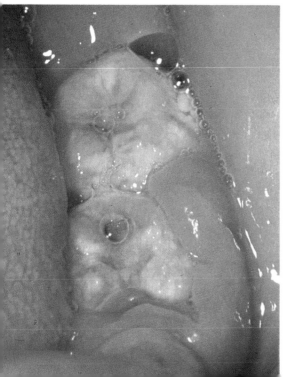

380 a What abnormality is seen in this female patient's mouth?

  b Which three causes would you consider?

381 This condition is drug-induced.
Which drugs may have been responsible?

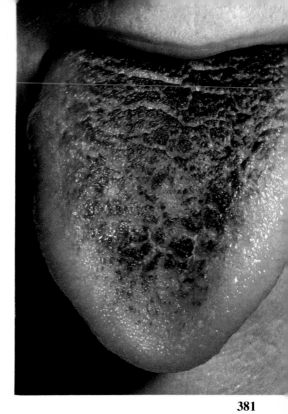

381

382 a What is the diagnosis?
  b What abnormalities are demonstrated?

382

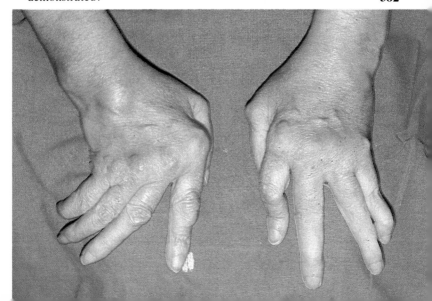

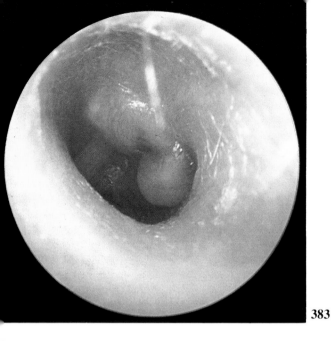

383

383 and 384 This twenty-two year old woman complained of a cough, fever and painful ear. Chest x-ray showed widespread patchy pulmonary infiltrates.

a What abnormality is shown
  i) in the blood film?
  ii) in the ear?
b What is the most likely diagnosis?
c What is the cause of the abnormality seen in the blood film?

384

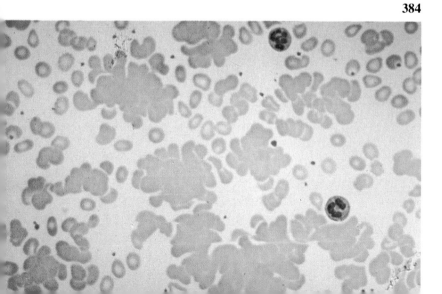

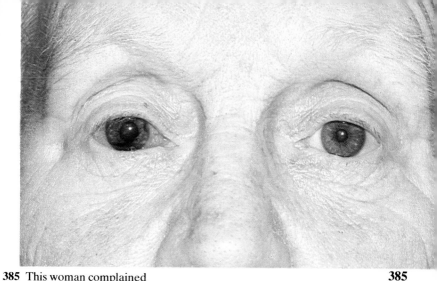

385 This woman complained
of a red eye and blurred
vision. There was no
history of trauma.
  a List four abnormalities
     present in the right eye.
  b Which diagnosis does
     this appearance
     suggest?

385

386

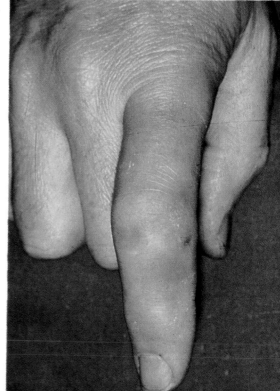

386 This man complains of a
painful forefinger of
several days duration. He
denies any history of
trauma.
  a What is the likely
     diagnosis?
  b Which occupational
     factors may be
     involved?
  c What is the appropriate
     treatment?

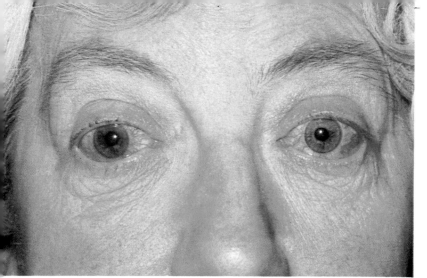

387 This woman complains of a roaring noise inside her head. **387**
    a What abnormalities are present?
    b What is the diagnosis?
    c What are the causes of this condition?

388

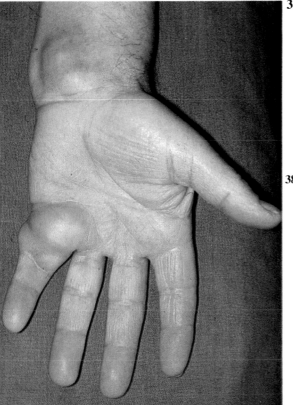

388 This patient has chronic renal failure. He has recently been found to have an early diastolic murmur audible along the left sternal border. His serum calcium is at the upper limit of normal; serum phosphate is greatly elevated.
    a What is the most likely nature of the hand abnormality seen?
    b How might this relate to his new murmur?

ANSWERS

The answers given below are necessarily brief as the aim of the series is to stimulate self-learning through further reading.

195 and 196
    a Subungual fibroma.
    b Phakoma.
    c Tuberose sclerosis.
    d 1 in 2 (usually autosomal dominant inheritance).

197 a Acromegaly.
    b i)   Pharmacological — bromocriptine.
        ii) Irradiation — external, trans-sphenoidal implant.
        iii) Surgery — transfrontal, trans-sphenoidal.
    c Degree of suprasellar extension, as assessed by CT scanning.

198 a 1 — Abdominal aorta.
        2 — Left adrenal tumour.
        3 — Right crus of diaphragm.
        4 — Top of right kidney.
        5 — Tip of spleen.
    b Left adrenal phaeochromocytoma. A Conn's tumour of this size is unlikely.

199 a Hyperinflation (elongated heart shadow; transverse upper ribs; anterior ends of seven ribs and posterior ends of eleven ribs visible in the lung fields).
    b Acute asthma.
    c Breathing in.

200 a Chronic myeloid (granulocytic) leukaemia.
    b i)   Cytogenetic analysis for Philadelphia chromosome.
        ii) Neutrophil alkaline phosphatase score (always low).
        iii) Vitamin B12 and B12 binding protein (characteristically elevated).
    c i)   Busulphan.
        ii) Allopurinol.
        iii) 6-mercaptopurine.
        iv) Thioguanine.
        v) Hydroxyurea.
        vi) Dibromomannitol.

201 a Progressive scarring with symblepharon formation leads to loss of vision in one third of sufferers.

b Deposition of IgG, IgA, and complement at the dermo-epidermal junction.

c No.

202 a Acute inferior myocardial infarction.

b Never. In the United Kingdom, his heavy goods vehicle licence will be revoked.

203 a Ectopic ACTH secretion from a carcinoma resulting in Cushing's syndrome.

b Oat cell carcinoma of bronchus most commonly. Other sites include thymus, pancreas, and thyroid. Bronchial carcinoid tumours may secrete ACTH.

c Hypokalaemic alkalosis.

d Plasma cortisol and ACTH are usually markedly elevated and show no suppression by dexamethasone nor metyrapone. Plain chest x-ray may show bronchial carcinoma or carcinoid. CT scanning may reveal smaller tumours in the thorax or abdomen.

204 a Femoral arterial embolism.

b Left atrium.

c Atrial fibrillation (although systemic embolisation in these circumstances typically follows alteration in rhythm).

205 a Tibial pseudofractures (Looser zones).

b Pubic and ischial rami.
Scapulae (axillary border).
Femoral and humeral necks.
Ribs.

c Osteomalacia.

206 a Scabies.

b Most commonly found on the sides of fingers, flexor aspects of wrist, sole of the foot.
(Also, elbows, buttocks, axillae).

c i) Isolation of female *Sarcoptes Scabei* from skin burrows.

ii) Skin biopsy (only occasionally necessary).

207 a Ventricular septal defect.

b (Intermittent) shunt reversal (right to left).

c i) Right and left ventricular pressures approximately equal.

ii) Pulmonary artery and aortic systolic pressures equal.

iii) Pulmonary artery diastolic pressure raised (but less than aortic diastolic).

iv) Minimal or absent step-up in oxygen saturation at ventricular level.

208 a Dermatitis herpetiformis.
   b Gluten-sensitive enteropathy.
   c i) Gluten free diet (skin lesions may occasionally remit on this alone).
     ii) Dapsone.

209 a Sycosis barbae
     (a deep folliculitis of the beard area).
   b Staphylococcus aureus.
   c The patient's own nose.

210 a Leukoplakia.
   b A pre-malignant condition.

211 a Failure of abduction of left eye.
   b Left abducens (VIth) nerve palsy.

212 a i) Cullen's sign (discolouration around the umbilicus).
     ii) Grey Turner's sign (flank discolouration).
   b i) Leaking aortic aneurysm.
     ii) Acute pancreatitis.

213 a i) Dupuytren's contractures.
     ii) Palmar erythema.
   b Alcoholic liver disease.
   c i) White nails.
     ii) Finger clubbing (more typically seen in primary biliary cirrhosis).
     iii) Spider naevi.
     iv) Jaundice.
     v) Tremor (of alcohol withdrawal, and of hepatic failure).

214 Retinal tear with retinal detachment.

215 a Apparent hypertrophy of the calf muscles.
   b Duchenne muscular dystrophy is most likely; Becker-type muscular dystrophy (also X-linked, but less severe) and myotonia congenita (rare) are also possible diagnoses.
   c Gower's sign.

216 and 217
     a i) Alopecia totalis, facial telangiectasia.
       ii) Cutaneous calcification, resorption of distal phalanges.
     b C.R.(E).S.T. syndrome. (Calcinosis, Raynaud's, (Esophageal dysmotility), Scleroderma, Telangiectasia).

218 a Ring forms of Plasmodium falciparum in erythrocytes.
   b Quinine intravenously or orally depending on the clinical status of the patient.
   c A combination preparation such as pyrimethamine with dapsone, or pyrimethamine with sulfadoxine.

219 a i) Spina bifida.
  ii) Bilateral hydroureter and hydronephrosis.
  iii) Ileal conduit (with ileostomy).
  iv) Congenital dislocation of the left hip.
b Hyperchloraemia; bicarbonate depletion.
c No.

220 a Chronic lymphocytic leukaemia.
b i) Haemolytic anaemia.
  ii) Hepatic infiltration.
  iii) Biliary duct obstruction secondary to lymphadenopathy at the porta hepatis.
c There is an initial rise before the count falls.

221 a Pinguecula.
b None. Surgery may be considered if there is marked disfigurement.

222 and 223
a Diffuse reticulonodular shadowing, consistent with interstitial lung disease.
b Single lytic lesion, with scalloped edge and no sclerotic reaction.
c Eosinophilic granuloma (histiocytosis X).

224 a Dermatitis artefacta (cigarette burns).
b Any part of the body accessible to the hands (typically face, and non-dominant hand and arm).

225 a Olecranon bursa.
b i) Demonstration of fluctuation.
  ii) Transillumination.

226 and 227
a i) Sparseness of haustral markings through most of the colon.
  ii) Narrowing of the distal sigmoid.
  iii) Ulceration.
  iv) Pseudopolyps.
  v) Loss of mucosal pattern.
b Ulcerative colitis.
c Pyoderma gangrenosum.
d i) Crohn's disease.
  ii) Rheumatoid arthritis (and some other arthritides, including Behçet's disease).
  iii) Myeloma/other monoclonal gammopathies.

228 and 229
a Bacterial endocarditis.
b The patient's own gastrointestinal tract.
c It is exquisitely sensitive to penicillin unlike most enteral streptococci.
d There is an increased incidence of colonic carcinoma in streptococcus bovis endocarditis.

230 a Kaposi's varicelliform eruption (eczema herpeticum or vaccinatum).
 b Vaccinia or herpes simplex virus.
 c Pre-existing skin disease, most commonly atopic eczema.
 Occasionally other inflammatory dermatoses may be responsible.

231 a Widespread cellulitis of the calf; ulceration superior to the medial malleolus; ascending lymphangitis.
 b Streptococcus pyogenes.
 c Stasis ulceration at the ankle allowing a portal of entry.

232 Fat embolism, following femoral shaft fracture.

233 a Winged left scapula.
 b Serratus anterior.
 c Long thoracic nerve palsy: in this case secondary to brachial plexus involvement by apical lung tumour. (Long thoracic nerve arises from 5th, 6th and 7th cervical roots).

234 a Relapsing polychondritis.
 b i) Sparing of non-cartilaginous tissue eg. lobules of the ear.
 ii) Increased urinary mucopolysaccharide excretion during exacerbations.
 c i) Aortitis with aortic regurgitation.
 ii) Laxity of epiglottis, tracheal and bronchial rings.

235 a Blue line (Burton's line) on gums.
 b Chronic lead poisoning.
 c i) Anaemia.
 ii) Peripheral motor neuropathy.
 iii) Encephalopathy.
 iv) Arthritis ('saturnine gout').

236 a Hypothyroidism.
 b Thyroxine replacement.

237 Laser burns.

238 and 239
 a Behçet's disease.
 b The eye usually completes the triad but the joints, central nervous system, colon, skin and vascular tree may be involved.
 c None.
 d Men.

240 a Risus sardonicus.
 b Tetanus.
 c i) Phenothiazines.
 ii) Metoclopramide.

241 a Gouty tophi.
    b i)   Serum uric acid.
      ii)   Compensated polarised light microscopy of expressed tophaceous material, (or of joint aspirate during an acute episode).

242 a Panhypopituitarism — craniopharyngioma.
                                    pituitary tumour.
    b i)   Skull x-ray.
      ii)   Computed tomography head scan.
      iii) Insulin hypoglycaemia — measure adrenocorticotrophic hormone, growth hormone and cortisol response.
      iv) Thyrotrophin stimulation test — thyroid stimulating hormone and prolactin response.
      v)   Gonadotrophin stimulation tests — response of luteinising hormone and follicle stimulating hormone to gonadotrophin releasing hormone stimulation.

243 a Erythema nodosum.
    b i)   Sarcoidosis.
      ii)   Reactive arthritis.
           eg. following gut infection with yersinia (pasteurella), salmonella, campylobacter jejunae.
      iii) Other enteropathic arthritis — in association with inflammatory bowel disease (Crohn's, ulcerative colitis).
      iv) Rheumatic fever.
      v)   Other uncommon possibilities include tuberculosis, polyarteritis nodosa, lepromatous leprosy, coccidioidomycosis.

244 and 245
    a Keratitis (interstitial).
    b Opaque material (injected bismuth) projected over both iliac crests.
    c Congenital syphilis.

246 a Disseminated choroiditis. (The pigmentation is racial).
    b i)   Syphilis (congenital or acquired).
      ii)   Tuberculosis.

247 a Norwegian scabies.
    b Sarcoptes scabiei hominis (— the same mite causes common human scabies. In Norwegian scabies the host response is impaired or modified).
    c i)   Mental deficiency.
      ii)   Immunodeficiency (including immunosuppressive drug therapy).
      iii) Diabetes mellitus.

248 and 249
    a i)   Swelling right thigh (with 'bowed' appearance).
      ii)   Venous distension right thigh.
      iii) Muscle wasting left thigh.

iv) Biopsy scar right thigh.
b i) Thickening and disordered bone formation typical of Paget's disease.
ii) Periosteal elevation with 'sun-ray' spiculation.
c Paget's disease.
d Osteosarcomatous change.

250 a Vitiligo.
b i) Diabetes mellitus.
ii) Autoimmune thyroid disease — thyroiditis, "idiopathic" hypothyroidism, Graves' disease, — also to less extent non-toxic goitre and thyroid carcinoma.
iii) Addison's disease.
iv) Other less common endocrine disorders — idiopathic hypopituitarism, autoimmune hypoparathyroidism.

251 a Symmetrical tongue enlargement.
b Acromegaly.

252 and 253
a i) Low hairline.
ii) Soft tissue swelling (in fact, lymphoedema).
b Turner's syndrome (45XO).

254 a No; the configuration of the chest leads establishes this to be true dextrocardia.
b Kartagener's syndrome.
c Chronic sinusitis; infertility.

255 a It is uncommon in women.
b Pigmentation is predominantly due to melanin deposition in the dermis.
c It is HLA linked; the HLA type varies in different affected families though breeds true within affected families.
d i) Carbohydrate tolerance improves.
ii) Cardiac failure is ameliorated.
iii) The risk of hepatoma is unchanged unless venesection is commenced before cirrhosis has begun to develop.

256 a Periventricular calcification.
b Epiloia (tuberose sclerosis).
c Rhabdomyoma.

257 a Retinitis pigmentosa.
b Abetalipoproteinaemia.
c Sensory ataxia due to posterior column degeneration is the commonest symptom. Other symptoms include muscular weakness, night blindness and ocular paresis.
d Alpha-tocopherol (vitamin E) may prevent or significantly retard the onset of neuropathy.

258 a i) Widespread nodular opacities in both lung fields.
ii) Trachea deviated to the right by neck mass.
b Thyroid carcinoma with lung metastases.

259 and 260
i) Pustular psoriasis (with psoriatic arthropathy).
ii) Reiter's syndrome.

261 a i) Failure of abduction of right eye — right VIth cranial nerve palsy.
ii) Dilated right pupil — suggesting right IIIrd cranial nerve palsy.
b i) Head or maxillofacial injury: direct nerve damage (rather than secondary to rising intracranial pressure, since the patient is fully conscious).
ii) Neurosurgery with pre-existing cranial nerve damage (eg lesion in the region of the cavernous sinus).
iii) Neurosurgery with cranial nerve damage at operation.

262 Down's syndrome (trisomy 21).

263 Acute rheumatic carditis (Carey-Coombs mitral murmur). The rash is of erythema marginatum, most typically seen on the trunk.

264 a Hidradenitis suppuritiva.
b None — no organism is consistently isolated.

265 a Sinus tachycardia; P pulmonale; right axis deviation; right ventricular hypertrophy.
b Cor pulmonale.

266 a i) Trisomy 21.
ii) Mongol mosaicism (46, XY/47, XY, + 21).
b i) Non-dysjunction.
ii) 'De novo' translocation.
iii) Familial translocation.

267 a Intracranial calcification — in curvilinear paired parallel lines.
b Sturge Weber syndrome.
c Other causes of calcification in this area include
i) Tuberose sclerosis.
ii) Congenital toxoplasmosis, cytomegalovirus infection.
iii) Angioma.
iv) Glioma (oligodendroglioma, astrocytoma).
v) Old haematoma.

268, 269 and 270
a i) Proptosis, conjunctival injection.
ii) Finger clubbing.
iii) 'Pretibial' myxoedema (in this case, in post tibial distribution).
b Graves' (or von Basedow's) disease.

271 a Discoid lupus erythematosus.
 b Erythema, scaling, follicular plugging, healing with atrophy, loss of pigment, telangiectasia and scarring.
 c About 5%.

272 a External angular dermoid.
 b It is a congenital lesion due to inclusion of ectodermal elements at sites of ectodermal fusion.
 c In all four quadrants of the orbit. In descending order of frequency: upper outer, upper inner, lower inner, lower outer.

273 a Pulmonary oedema.
 b Rupture of the anterior papillary muscle causing acute mitral regurgitation or perforation of the interventricular septum.

274 a A superficial papillomatous tumour of the soft palate.
 b Squamous carcinoma.
 c Tobacco smoking or chewing; heavy alcohol consumption; severe iron deficiency anaemia especially in women; syphilis.

275, 276, 277 and 278
 Patient 1 — Dermatitis herpetiformis.
 Patient 2 — Pemphigoid.
 Patient 3 — Epidermolysis bullosa (dominant dystrophic form).
 Patient 4 — Pemphigus vulgaris.

279 and 280
 a i) Toxic shock syndrome (TSS).
  ii) Toxic epidermal necrolysis (TEN).
 b Exotoxin producing staphylococci.
 c The toxins have different actions. They are produced by staphylococci of differing phage type.

281 a Myasthenia gravis.
 b Edrophonium chloride (Tensilon) test.
 c i) CT scanning of upper mediastinum (for thymoma).
  ii) Tests for associated autoimmune or connective tissue diseases. (e.g. systemic lupus erythematosus).
  iii) Antibodies to acetyl choline receptor, striated muscle.
  iv) Electromyography (± combined with Tensilon test).

282 a i) Pale, cloudy retina.
  ii) 'Cherry red' macula.
  iii) Fragmented arterial blood columns ('trucking') — seen in inferior nasal artery and branch of superior temporal artery.
 b Central retinal artery occlusion.
 c Yes.
 d Giant cell arteritis (cranial, temporal arteritis) — tongue and jaw claudication are said to be pathognomonic of this.

283 and 284
- a Xanthelasmata.
- b Carotene (her sclerae are white, therefore jaundice is unlikely).
- c i) Hypothyroidism.
  - ii) Diabetes mellitus.
  - iii) Familial hypercholesterolaemia.
  - iv) Primary biliary cirrhosis.
  - v) Nephrotic syndrome.

285 a No. It shows a bulky uterus.
- b A Gestation sac of approximately 6 weeks.
  - B Intrauterine contraceptive device.

286 a i) Umbilical hernia.
  - ii) Gynaecomastia.
- b 120 mls.
  - The 'Puddle Sign'. With the patient on "all fours" simultaneous percussion in the flank and auscultation around the most dependent part of the abdomen is carried out.
  - The presence of shifting dullness in the supine position generally indicates a litre or more of ascites. Demonstration of a fluid thrill is less sensitive.

287 a Periorbital oedema.
- b Anthrax.
- c Differential diagnosis includes staphylococcal infection, cow-pox, accidental vaccinia, cat scratch disease. Rarer causes include blastomycosis, sporotrichosis.
- d Yes. Untreated mortality may be as high as 20%

288 a Diffuse gastric mucosal irregularity.
- b 'Leather bottle stomach'; linitis plastica (diffuse adenocarcinoma).

289 a Blue rubber bleb naevus syndrome.
- b Haemangiomata of bowel (usually small intestinal).
- c Liver, spleen, central nervous system.

290 a Tinea cruris due to Trichophyton rubrum.
- b A topical antifungal such as miconazole, clotrimazole, or Whitfield's ointment, or systemic antifungal therapy with ketoconazole or griseofulvin.

291 a i) Multiple neurofibromata.
  - ii) Café-au-lait spots.
- b Von Recklinghausen's disease (neurofibromatosis).
- c Left acoustic neuroma.

292 a Lesch-Nyhan syndrome.
- b X-linked recessive.
- c Hypoxanthine-guanine phosphoribosyl transferase.

93 a Caput medusae.
    b Portal venous hypertension.
    c i)   Oesophageal varices.
       ii)   Acute gastric erosions.
       iii) Peptic ulceration.

94 and 295
    a Lid lag (Von Graeve's sign).
    b It is a useful sign of thyrotoxicosis (but can also be seen in marked anxiety and with sympathomimetic drug therapy).

96 and 297
    a i)   Subperiosteal resorption of the phalanges, and erosion of the terminal tufts.
       ii)   Scratch marks.
    b These suggest pre-existing chronic renal impairment (ie. acute-on-chronic uraemia).
    c 1.010.

98 and 299
    a Psoriatic arthropathy.
    b Chloroquine or hydroxychloroquine.

00 a Absent clavicles.
    b Cranio cleido dysostosis.
    c i)   Skull.
       ii)   Pubic symphysis.

301 a Clitoral hypertrophy.
     b Indicates significant increase in circulating androgens.

302 a Addison's disease.
     b Demonstration of an impaired cortisol response to 250 µg aqueous tetracosactrin given intramuscularly.
     c Eosinophilia; lymphocytosis.

303 a Neovascularisation.
     b Diabetes mellitus and sickle cell disease are the commonest causes. Others include hyperviscosity syndromes; sarcoidosis; Behçet's disease; Eales disease; exudative retinopathy.

304 No. The lack of skin creases indicates that it is less than thirty-six weeks gestation.

305 a Rupture of the long head of biceps.
     b There is usually no significant loss of power.
     c Repeated local injections of corticosteroids for bicipital tendonitis.

306 and 307
  a i)   Left pleural effusion.
    ii) Left pneumothorax.
    iii) Mediastinal shift to the left.
    iv) Surgical clips left upper zone (on stump of left upper lobe
         bronchus).
    v)   Pleural fluid/thickening right cardiophrenic angle.
  b Widespread nodular opacities in both lung fields.
  c Bronchial carcinoma with pulmonary metastases.
    (The upper film was taken shortly after thoracotomy for left upper
    lobectomy).

308   i)   Her 'normal' serum thyroxine (T4) may have been at the low end
               of the normal range. 148 nmol/l may therefore represent as much
               as a two-fold rise.
          ii) Isolated T3 (tri-iodothyronine) toxicosis.
          iii) Diminished concentration of thyroxine binding globulin (TBG).
               This may represent a normal variant; or may be secondary to
               thyrotoxicosis itself, nephrotic syndrome, or to an inherited,
               sex-linked deficiency in TBG. Drug-induced reduction in TBG
               (eg high dose corticosteroids, testosterone) is unlikely here, as is
               active acromegaly.
          iv) Displacement of T4 from TBG, increased degradation of T4 (both
               may occur with phenytoin therapy).
          v)   Euthyroidism — the clinical features may be those of anxiety.
          vi) Sampling or laboratory error.

309 1 True aortic lumen.
        2 False aortic lumen.
        3 Intimal flap of dissection.
        4 Right kidney with white cortex and darker medulla.
        5 Tip of right lobe of liver.

310 a Yes.
        b This is a kerion due to cattle ringworm, Trichophyton verrucosum.
        c Oral antifungal therapy (griseofulvin or ketoconazole) plus systemic
          antibiotic to eradicate bacterial superinfection.

311   i)   Mycobacterium tuberculosis.
          ii) Staphylococcus aureus.
          iii) Klebsiella pneumoniae.
          iv) Bacteroides (and other anaerobes).
          v)   Others include:
               Actinomycosis, histoplasmosis, coccidioidomycosis,
               aspergillosis, nocardiosis.

312 a Leptospirosis (Weil's disease).
        b Yes. Leptospirosis was formerly common in this group.
        c Rodents, particularly the brown rat in the United Kingdom.

313 a Cutaneous larva migrans (creeping eruption).
   b Ancylostoma brasiliense is the commonest cause but others include A. caninum, Strongyloides stercoralis, Necator americanus, and Gasterophilus.

314 VIIth nerve neuroma in association with neurofibromatosis. Pigmented 'café au lait' patches are seen on the trunk (in addition to an old biopsy scar in the neck).

315 a Acromegaly.
   b Median nerve compression (carpal tunnel syndrome).

316 a High myopic degeneration.
   b Long.

317 a Secondary syphilis.
   b Diffuse proliferative glomerulonephritis.

318   i)   Enlargement, erosion, and/or double floor of the pituitary fossa.
      ii) Enlargement of the frontal sinuses.
      iii) Increase in the angle of the mandible.
      iv) Prognathism.
      v)   Thickening of the cranial vault.

319 a Scurvy (Vitamin C deficiency).
   b No.
   c i)   Platelet ascorbic acid levels (plasma levels less helpful).
      ii) Ascorbic acid saturation test.

320 and 321
   a i)   Distended superficial veins. (The right chest has also been recently shaved, and radiotherapy markers are visible).
      ii) Large irregular opacity in the right upper zone; enlargement of right hilum and upper mediastinum.
   b Superior vena caval obstruction, secondary to bronchogenic carcinoma with massive mediastinal lymphadenopathy.
   c Radiotherapy.

322 a Fissuring of the lateral margins of the tongue.
   b Recurrent facial palsy.
   c Melkersson's syndrome.

323 a Air in the soft tissues.
   b Gas gangrene. (Infection with gas-forming organisms, eg clostridium perfringens).

324 a Osteogenesis imperfecta congenita (in this form, type III osteogenesis imperfecta, the sclerae are often white).
   b Hyperplastic callus formation (possibly in relation to fracture; not necessarily so).

325 a Benign melanoma of the choroid.
    b None, but the patient should be followed up with regular fundal photographs.

326 a Fixed drug eruption.
    b i) Tetracycline.
      ii) Sulphonamide (eg sulphamethoxazole, as in co-trimoxazole).
    c Oral challenge — lesion, once healed, will reappear two to three hours after ingestion of the offending drug. This does not carry a risk of anaphylaxis.
    (patch tests on involved skin give variable results; on uninvolved skin, patch testing is negative).

327 The ECG should be repeated at the correct voltage. It proves to be completely normal.

328 a Nodular prurigo.
    b None. Local infiltration with corticosteroid may be helpful, usually briefly.

329 a Hydatid disease (Echinococcosis).
    b Global.
    c Man is an accidental intermediate host.

330 a Oral candidiasis (thrush).
    b Broad-spectrum antibiotics; corticosteroids; immunosuppressive agents.

331 a Lumbar myelogram (using water-soluble contrast medium).
    b Lateral protrusion of the L5/S1 disc (right side).
    c i) Impaired sensation on the outer border of foot (including fourth and fifth toes) and sole (sparing the great toe).
      ii) Weakness is usually limited to the toe dorsiflexors (especially extensor hallucis longus).
      iii) Impaired or absent ankle jerk.

332 a Basal cell carcinoma (rodent ulcer).
    b No —
      i) Dissemination of basal cell carcinoma is uncommon (lymphatic dissemination more so).
      ii) Lymphatic drainage from post-auricular skin is not to the submandibular nodes (rather, to retroauricular and upper deep cervical nodes).

333 and 334
    a i) Hyperextensible joints.
      ii) 'Papyraceous' scar.
    b Ehlers Danlos syndrome.
    c Mitral valve prolapse ('floppy' mitral valve).

335 a Chloasma of pregnancy.

    b Breasts, linea alba (becoming linea nigra); occasionally in striae gravidarum.

336 a Pigmentation.

    b Addison's disease.

    c The development of Addison's disease must have been more than two - years ago.

337 and 338

    a Pulmonary actinomycosis.

    b None.

    c The source of infection is usually the mouth. The pulmonary infection is often due to aspiration. Poor oral hygiene is more typically related to cervicofacial actinomycosis.

339 a Periorbital cellulitis.

    b Non-fatal complications include,

        i)   Cavernous sinus thrombosis.

        ii)   Meningitis.

        iii) Brain abscess.

        iv) Optic atrophy.

    c Helpful signs include,

        i)   Impaired visual acuity.

        ii)   Pupillary defects.

        iii) Papilloedema.

        iv) Raised intraocular pressure.

340 a Shingles (herpes zoster).

    b Cervical 7 and 8.

341 a Acne rosacea.

    b i)   Conjunctivitis.

       ii)   Blepharitis.

       iii) Hordeolum (stye).

       iv) Keratitis.

342 a Left apical pneumothorax.

343 a Eyeball prosthesis.

    b He has metastatic malignant melanoma from choroidal melanoma (the affected eye having been enucleated).

344 a Erythroderma.

    b Chronic lymphatic leukaemia, Hodgkin's disease.

    c i)   Hypothermia.

       ii)   Infections — cutaneous, respiratory.

       iii) Thrombophlebitis.

       iv) Peripheral circulatory failure.

345 a Von Willebrand's disease.
   b It will be prolonged.
   c Normal aggregation to collagen.
   d 50% of boys.

346 a Mycetoma (Madura foot).
   b None. (Madura foot is caused by fungi and, occasionally, actinomycetes).
   c None.

347 No sign will reliably differentiate between the conditions.

348 a Scrofula.
   b Mycobacterium tuberculosis, though bovine or atypical mycobacteria may be causative.

349 and 350
   a Paget's disease.
   b Not necessarily: specific treatment is indicated if there is sensorineural impairment secondary to skull foraminal compression; more often, deafness in Paget's disease is due to involvement of the ossicles or to coincidental disease.

351 a Rheumatoid nodules.
   b Fibrous stroma containing granulomatous foci. Each granuloma consists of
      i)   A central zone of fibrinoid necrosis, containing cellular and nuclear debris, and fibrin.
      ii) A rim of fibroblasts and histiocytes arranged in palisades.
      iii) A surrounding chronic inflammatory infiltrate (plasma cells, lymphocytes, occasional giant cells).
   c Positive tests for rheumatoid factor (Rose Waaler, RA latex tests).

352 a Neck webbing.
   b Turner's syndrome.
   c Coarctation of the aorta.

353 and 354
      a i)   Choroiditis.
         ii) Intracerebral calcification.
      b Congenital toxoplasmosis.

355 a Staining of teeth due to tetracycline administration.
   b Tetracycline-stained teeth may fluoresce when viewed in ultra-violet light.
   c Differing rates of odontogenesis and calcification of individual teeth modify the amount of tetracycline taken up by the teeth.
   d No, in fact they are less prone than normal to caries.

356 a i)   Right mastectomy.
         ii) Local recurrence of breast carcinoma.

       iii) Oedema of the arm.

       iv) Radiation skin damage.

    b Cutaneous haemiangiosarcoma (Stewart-Treves syndrome).

357 a Imperforate anus; meconium issuing from the urethra.

     b Rectovesical or rectourethral fistula.

358 a Embolism of mural thrombus from the left ventricle. A recent anterior myocardial infarction is seen on the ECG.

     b Yes, unless there is a contraindication. There have been no adequate clinical studies to determine the optimal time to anticoagulate such patients, but delayed anticoagulation is associated with a higher incidence of recurrent embolism.

     c Mural thrombus may be detected by two-dimensional echocardiography, contrast ventriculography, or radionucleide scanning.

359 a Carbuncle.

     b Diabetes mellitus.

360 and 361

     a Erythema multiforme.

     b Organisms include herpes simplex, mycoplasma pneumoniae, chlamydiae, orf and streptococci.

     c No, though they may help differentiate it from diseases such as pemphigoid if there is doubt.

362 a Prolapse of a tumour mass into the left ventricle.

     b Left atrial myxoma (with systemic embolisation).

     c Cardiac surgery, as soon as possible.

363 Femoral arterial blood sampling for blood gas analysis.

364 a Bilateral pitting arm oedema.

     b Superior vena caval obstruction.

     c Lymphoma, especially Hodgkin's.

     d Massive upper mediastinal lymphadenopathy.

365 a i) Plantar erythema.

       ii) Trophic ulcer.

     b Alcohol — causing liver disease and peripheral sensory neuropathy. (Diabetes mellitus and vasculitic rheumatoid arthritis are less likely possibilities).

366 a Microaneurysms, dot haemorrhages and hard exudates.

     b i) Urinalysis for glucose.

       ii) Plasma glucose: fasting, postprandial or as part of an oral glucose tolerance test.

367 and 368
    a Band keratopathy.
    b Swelling of right shoulder (due to subcutaneous calcification).
    c Tertiary hyperparathyroidism.

369 a 'Fresh' striae (atrophicae).
    b Cushing's syndrome.
    c They cannot be discriminated with certainty. Distribution,
       appearance and histology may be the same.

370 a None. The epiphysis of the tubercle is beginning to ossify but this
       appearance is normal.
    b Osteochondritis of the tibial apophysis (Osgood — Schlatter's
       disease).
    c None. Restriction of excessive physical activity or occasionally a
       walking long leg plaster may be suggested.

371 and 372
    a Spina bifida occulta.
    b Diastematomyelia — with linear growth, stretching of tethered cord
       and nerve roots across fibrous septum leads to nerve root damage and
       splitting of the cord.

373 and 374
    a Arthritis mutilans.
    b Rheumatoid arthritis.
    c i)   Periarticular soft tissue swelling.
       ii) Periarticular osteoporosis.
       iii) Joint space narrowing.

375, 376, 377 and 378
    a Facioscapulohumeral muscular dystrophy.
    b i)   Weak tibialis anterior.
       ii) Impaired biceps, triceps reflexes. Supinator, knee and ankle jerks
           normal.
    c i)   Orbicularis oris, serratus anterior.
       ii) Left pectoralis major (which is absent).
    d Life expectancy is usually normal.

379 a He is haemophiliac. A.I.D.S. may be transmissable in blood
       products.
    b Male homosexuals and their contacts.
       Heroin addicts.
       Haitians.

380 a Gum hyperplasia/hypertrophy/infiltration.
    b i)   Phenytoin (in association with bacterial plaque).
       ii) Normal pregnancy (and oral contraceptives).
       iii) Acute myelomonocytic leukaemia.

381 i) Oral penicillins.
ii) Other topical oral antibiotics and mouthwashes (eg. sodium perborate).
iii) Bismuth.

382 a Rheumatoid arthritis.
b i) Ulnar deviation and prominent metacarpal heads (subluxation at MCP joints).
ii) Boutonniere (index left) and swan neck (5th left) deformities.
iii) Extensor tendon nodules.
iv) Wasting of dorsal interossei.
(This patient also has ruptured 3rd, 4th and 5th extensor tendons on the right with prominent right ulnar styloid).

383 and 384
a i) Red cell agglutination.
ii) Bullous myringitis.
b Mycoplasma pneumoniae infection.
c Cold agglutination occurs due to the development of a macroglobulin (IgM) directed against I antigen on the red cell surface.

385 a i) Hyphaema.
ii) Conjunctival suffusion.
iii) Irregular, dilated pupil.
iv) Depression of the iris at the limbus in the three o'clock position.
b The abnormalities of the iris and pupil in the absence of trauma suggest a tumour of the ciliary body, most likely a malignant melanoma. (The iris appearance should not be mistaken for an iridectomy, which is unlikely at this site).

386 a Erysipeloid due to cutaneous infection by Erysipelothrix rhusiopathiae.
b It is most commonly seen in abbatoir or fish workers.
c The organism is sensitive to penicillins, cephalosporins, erythromycin, tetracyclines, and chloramphenicol.

387 a i) Bilateral exophthalmos.
ii) Conjunctival injection.
b Carotico-cavernous fistula.
c Spontaneous rupture of an infraclinoid aneurysm into the cavernous sinus; traumatic following skull fracture (particularly basitemporal fracture) or neurosurgery.

388 a Subcutaneous calcification.
b Metastatic calcification in the aortic valve may have led to aortic incompetence.

INDEX